THE

FAT

DEMONS

Grace Publishing
Memphis, Tennessee 38109

All scripture references taken from the King James Version, unless otherwise indicated.

Grace Publishing is a Ministry of Abundant Grace Fellowship
843 West Raines Road Memphis, Tennessee 38109
901-789-GRACE (4722), or 877-88-GRACE
Senior Pastor, Dwayne N. Hunt
www.dwaynehunt.com
First printing, 1999
Reprints available — write, call or fax
www.drmarlenehunt.com

The FAT Demons

Printed in the USA by

MP
MORRIS PUBLISHING

3212 East Highway 30 • Kearney, NE 68847 • 1-800-650-7888

**Dedi-
cation:
This book
is sure to bless.
Loving thanks to my husband,
Pastor Dwayne Hunt
For enduring the
Spiritual Ugly
As this
Book
Came
Forth
Into
Print.**

CONTENTS:

The Fat
of the Land

My daddy is an Old Testament man who would read the Bible out loud for hours at a time. He no doubt, read about the *fat* of the land. Daddy didn't have a concordance, or Hebrew-Greek dictionary, so as he read, he understood fat to mean *fat*. An old fashioned Baptist, Daddy didn't have the *concordance* of the Holy Spirit either, so he understood fat to mean *fat*. At meal time, Daddy's plates were fuller than anyone's. Mom is an excellent cook, but it was as though Daddy was trying to eat the *fat of the land* that he read about in the scriptures. We'd ask, *"Daddy, don't you think you're getting big?"*

He would reply, adjusting his pants back above his *dunlap, "I'm prosperous."*

Now that we have read the Bible for ourselves, we understand more. Daddy was brought up during the Great Depression; and was taught to eat all of his food, *when he had food.* That clean-your-plate mentality carried over to adulthood. And when added to what he read, became a confirmation for Daddy to *eat.* Being fat *in the old days,* was a sign of prosperity, but being thin was a sign of poverty. Considering the dearth of food during the Depression, and believing that *fat* meant prosperous, Daddy ate abundantly, to prove he was no longer poor.

Fat still means fat, but now we have Hebrew-Greek dictionaries, concordances, and revelation through the Holy Spirit, to help us understand the different *kinds* of Old Testament fat. There was the fat of animals, the fat of man, and the fat of the land. The *fat of the land* is the prosperity, abundance, spoils, resources, and harvest of the actual land. When God says you can eat the fat, He means partake, or use.

Almost all of the Old Testament fat is metaphorical; not literal. God is not saying to eat fat, and get physically heavy.

And take your father and your households, and come unto me: and I will give you the good of the land of Egypt, and ye shall eat the fat of the land. (Gen 45:18)

The Sacrifice of Fat

*W*hile there is much talk about fat in the Old Testament, the word, *fat* is not even in the New Testament. Why? Could it be with the birth of Jesus, that fat became obsolete? Oh, were it so. But in a sense, it is true. The sacrifice of animals was practically an everyday thing for Old Testament people, but things changed drastically by the time of the New Testament. Animal sacrifice was common under the Old Covenant, so God told man exactly how to handle the meat, blood, and fat of the ritual.

And the priest shall burn them upon the altar: it is the food of the offering made by fire for a sweet savour: all the fat is the LORD's.
It shall be a perpetual statute for your generations throughout all your dwellings, that ye eat neither fat nor blood. (Lev 3:16-17)

The eating of the sacrificial fat was as abominable as the eating of blood; the *life* was considered to be in the blood, therefore ingesting it was strictly forbidden. The fat was delicacy; it was the Lord's, and not to be eaten. Eating marbled steaks, or roasts that had fat in them, was fine, as long as they were prepared for food. But the suet, the fat of the sacrificed animal, was entirely the Lord's. To eat of the Lord's portion of a sacrifice was a religious violation punishable swiftly, and severely.

Speak unto the children of Israel, saying,
Ye shall eat no manner of fat,
of ox, or of sheep, or of goat. (Lev 7:23)

If the animal was not killed, but died on it's own, then no part of it should be eaten.

And the fat of the beast that dieth of itself, and the fat
of that which is torn with beasts, may be used in any
other use: but ye shall in no wise eat of it. (Lev 7:23-24).

**The Bible has everything,
even the rules for Road Kill.**

There may not be any talk of fat in the New Testament, because the animal sacrifice became obsolete by
the once and for all sacrifice of the Lamb of God, Jesus
Christ.

But this man, after he had offered one sacrifice for sins
for ever, sat down on the right hand of God; (Heb 10:12)

Thank God, in the Better Covenant, there are no more
animal sacrifices. But does that mean we should eat as
much of anything, as we want? No. You'd never see an
All You Can Eat sign at an Old Testament sacrificial
service, or Holy Communion. Those are the services designed to truly give God honor.

How can we, in the times in which we live, stop overeating, especially on *feast* holidays, and honor God?
Here's how: the Old Testament sacrifice of fat doesn't
have to be an old sacrifice any more. Just as we offer

the sacrifice of Praise, or the sacrifice of our offerings, why not offer God the sacrifice of *fat*, once again. Eating no meat or dairy products would be a true sacrifice; offer Him the delicacy, offer God the best.

The Sacrifice of Fat:
Fast fat for a week, or a month and see how it pleases God, and blesses you.

(Consult your physician before beginning any diet or exercise program. Some fatty acids are essential for good health; a long-term fast that reduces fat, instead of eliminating fat completely, can also be very beneficial.)

The Fat of the Man

The murder of Eglon, the King of Moab, was the first talk of physical fat in the Bible. Eglon's fat was so profuse, that when he was stabbed, the dagger that was thrust in him, *stuck*! Why we are told this story is left to your interpretation; but that's a lot of fat.

> ... and Eglon was a very fat man.
> ... Ehud ... took the dagger ...and thrust it into his belly:
> And the haft also went in after the blade; and the fat
> closed upon the blade, so that he could not draw the
> dagger out of his belly; ... (Judges 3:17, and 22-23)

The Bible warns of overeating and lustful appetites. Eglon may have been a man with a hedonistic appetite. We are given Eglon as the example of a worldly king who oppressed Israel, and gave in to his own lusts. On the opposite end, is Eli, the priest. Eli was a man of God, but he ate to become a very heavy man. **Food does not discriminate, so the man must.** It does not matter if you are in the world, or saved, overeating will add fat. Proverbs 23:2, warns that the man that eats too much, should take a knife to his own throat. Eli's death didn't involve a knife; when he heard of the word of the ark of the covenant, he died in a fall. God's judgements are spiritual, they don't necessarily have to do with a person's size, or weight.

> **... he fell from off the seat backward by the side of the gate, and his neck brake, and he died: for he was an old man, and heavy.... (1 Sam 4:18)**
> (This is where the term *keeled over dead* comes from.)

If Eli hadn't been so big, his fall, though a response to a spiritual matter, may not have been fatal. Eating a lot doesn't prove prosperity, help agility, or increase lifespan. And if the *why* and *how* of eating is not understood, food may be a route for demonic entrance, footholds, traps, or snares. Fatal or non-fatal *falls* can result in the spiritual, or physical realm, from food, and misuse of it. Food can be the cause of addictions, and death.

The root of many of man's troubles, problems, and curses is **food.** An obedient Adam and Eve, in the Garden, would not have eaten of the Tree. But while under the temptation of the actual devil, if they had *fasted*, neither would have fallen into sin.

When Jesus was in the wilderness for 40 days and nights, He was personally tempted of the devil, (like Adam and Eve), except **Jesus won!** Jesus was *fasting; was that a coincidence?* **No!** God's kingdom doesn't work by accident, or chance; Jesus did not stumble, or happen into ministry. Jesus did not *happen* to be fasting at the time He was tempted. He was showing us how to overcome, even in times of temptation.

The first part of Jesus' temptation was the offer of food. Why would the devil offer food, unless there was something to it? Why do you *bless* food before eating? Is there something in food, about food, or about the eating of food, that needs to be *blessed* before consumption? Probably. When asking grace, you thank God, and ask that the food is both nourishing and *safe* to eat. You mean physically safe; hoping that the food will not make you sick, or kill you. *We should add* **spiritually** **safe***. If we considered the spiritual, as we should, we wouldn't eat a lot of things that we eat.*

Food, spiritual? Yes. Why do you pray over what you eat? And if your physical body is being used for spiritual works, godly works, then what you put in it, how you treat it, is very important. When you care about something you take care of it. If you want something to last a long time, you take care of it. Spiritually, you want to last a long time. To have authority in the earth, you need a physical body. To exert yourself spiritually in the earth, you need a physical body. To exert yourself effectively, you need a healthy, and fit, body. Dead men don't sing, and sick men aren't as effective in ministry as healthy men.

While food gives natural strength; look at Popeye's power-spinach-rush. Our God confounds the wise; how does a **fasting man** have *more spiritual strength* than a man who eats? If Jesus had eaten, in that first tempta- tion, He would have been spiritually weakened, rather than strong. And thank God, He didn't; after the first temptation, especially when spiritually weak. Am I saying the spiritually weak over eat? If food is a temptation to you, and you overeat, then you are weak. When giving in to one temptation, the next temptation would have been easy as cake, (or pie). After eating everything on the table, eating the pie or cake is easy.

> **If you are under temptation,
> or feel you are about to enter temptation,
> consider fasting.**

Party Over Here!

An old TV ad claims you *can make friends with Koolaid.* Food and, or beverage often accompanies social invitations, and events. Sometimes the food *is* the entertainment. When socializing, (eating especially), believing to be among friends, guards are let down. Consider how the prophets eating at Jezebel's table, (1 King 18:19), did her bidding. Many business deals are made over meals. Mafia movies depict bad things happening in restaurants, and at dinner tables, as the victims dine. When it comes to attack, ambush, and deception, eating is one of the ultimate distractions. There is a certain kind of power associated with food; when planning a party, which is made first, the menu, or the guest list? Depends on what you want to accomplish, right?

Many parties start with food, then escalate to things such as alcohol or drugs. If you told someone you were having a drug party, who would come? Okay, I asked that. One enemy trick is to bring out alcohol and drugs, after the party crowd has gathered. Luke 15:23 invites the eating of food, and the making of merry, which is **to party**. That passage in Luke was about something good;

but combined with something bad, (food with drugs, for example), an old devil trick is exposed. *A spoonful of sugar, helps the medicine go down.* The food is the sugar, something you know and like, but it's deception, when the *medicine,* is not really medicine.

Food is necessary for life. Thankfully, God has promised us all things that pertain to life and godliness, (2 Peter 1:3), and He provides in abundance. In our culture, we have the luxury of eating three, or more, times a day. These can be times of temptation, if something bad is tied to the activity. If the eating is done improperly, or mishandled, deception can be slipped in more easily than just offering something bad alone. Free food can be found at *happy hours*, where alcoholic beverages are sold. You'll find food at gambling events; and extremely cheap, or even free food at casinos. For store-owners' convenience, food courts are in the mall. You don't ever have to go home; you are encouraged to stay all day; use up all your free time, and overspend while you're at it. Besides having the luxury of regular meals, we are bombarded with food temptations, almost everywhere we go.

I recently saw fresh popcorn vending in a courts building— as if court is entertainment! Complete food courts *in* state and municipal courts buildings are sure to be next. *(I'm prophesying).* There's a large crowd of people, they can't leave until their number is called, they are stressed out, nervous, and worried, (conditions under which many eat). Most left home in a hurry, without eating. Food courts, even in such an odd place, carries a big potential for making money. Don't be surprised when you see it come to pass.

Talk about a party! Sodom and Gomorrah, which is well-known for sex perversions, had more *food* than realized. Don't joke that when certain kinds of men get together, they cook and decorate. It's no joking matter; the *spirit of sexual perversion, the one responsible for male or female homosexuality, is the same spirit that leads to the sexual molestation and abuse of **children.*** In many cases, the spiritual *transference* happens to a child at the time of the molestation.

But guess what, that spirit really influences *eating*. Other than eating, there may be nothing innocent about this bold, and *perverse spirit*. This spirit, like too many others, influences man to the lusts of the flesh; to live life to the fullest; whatever that *fullest* may be. Many U.S. cities are known for culinary excellence, *and* homosexual populations. There's eating, drinking, partying, and sex — of all kinds; which many consider, "living it up". By tying food and perverse sexual behavior, I am **not** saying that all male chefs are homosexual; anymore than a woman who *doesn't* cook is gay, but lusts for food, and sexual perversion, (including, but not limited to homo-sexuality), are often found together, just as they were in Sodom and Gomorrah, (Gen. 18 & 19).

Fulfilling an exaggerated lust for food, on a large scale, has often been the indication of the beginning of the end of many civilizations. Our society is exhibiting characteristics similar to the declining Roman Empire, which had just about every flesh desire fulfilled. Polyg-amy, concubines, and harems were legal; men had as many women as they wanted. But they wanted more, different, strange, and *perverted.* They even built homo-sexual bath houses. Fulfilling the lust for food, and flesh pleasures, they hosted feasts, banquets, and orgies which lasted days, on end. They ate while reclining, as the Empire was declining.

Christians were publicly fed to lions, or gladiators fought them, unfairly to the death. Christians were not in style, *they were the entertainment*, being sacrificed regu-larly, (before the time of Emperor Constantine).

Where there is entertainment, there is food. Count on it. If you see food, no matter what's going on, the people believe what they are doing is:

- Okay, acceptable, or all right.
- Entertainment, no matter how wrong it is.

To a Roman, a barbarian didn't know Greek philosophy, and what implement to use at the dining table. And the world still judges by the outward. Avid Christians are still considered fanatics. You can see how the world we live in is very much the same — it's all about parties, wild sex, and ministering to the flesh. It's all about now, and today; most people aren't thinking about eternity. Unfortunately, the worldly man is *still* only looking at the outward, and he still wants the same things as ever: food, sex, parties, fun, prosperity, creature comforts, and flesh desires. Like Jesus, we disciples, must still witness to the unsaved, no matter what their spiritual flaws, sinful desires, lack of communication, or level of understanding may be.

But because the things of God are spiritually understood, and the world does not have God's Spirit, communication may be strained, or understanding may be lacking, between the saved and unsaved. We Christians must still practice our faith, and witness to others; it's the Great Commission, (Acts 1:8). We cannot fail to share the Gospel with others. Don't give up on people — not even those with the hardest of hearts. Remember, there was a time when you didn't have God's Spirit. You may not have been a murderer, or a hater, or maybe you were, but look how far you've come, because of God's love and grace.

Because of God's Spirit, your understanding has been

opened, (Eph 1:18). You are, or are becoming, more spiritually aware, and alert to deception. Caution: Food can still be one such deception. To date, many books have been written about foods as aphrodisiacs; purporting that food can get you sex, (wining and dining), and certain foods, (oysters), are said to enhance sexual enjoyment. If this is true, then has food been used *on you,* as an aphrodisiac, or as a tool to lull you into a false sense of comfort?

Women are taught as girls, *the way to a man's heart is through his stomach.* After eating, blood flows to the stomach. As digestion begins, sleepiness, dullness, or extreme relaxation may follow; awareness decreases, and laziness may increase. Stomach-consciousness may increase—(thinking about how you feel, instead of what's happening around you.) One may be more prone to suggestion, *(Why don't we get married?);* or more easily influenced, *(Honey, I want a new car).*

You may be fed so you can then be led, *(Let's go to the mall.)* If you fed a dog, or a cat, it will follow you almost anywhere. You've heard the saying: *There is no free lunch*; are you being fed for a reason? Something happens when folks are fed, guards are let down, loyalties are formed, and deals are made. The devil knows this — careful. In the world, everyone who feeds you may not be a friend.

Are you being fed so you can be led?

This does not mean don't eat with people; nor does it mean don't accept invitations that involve food. It does not mean that people perceive your invitations in a negative way, necessarily. This only means in any situation, use wisdom and discernment. Don't let food, and the offers of food deceive you into thinking that everything is okay, or as it should be, especially when you think the person inviting you wants something from you, that you wouldn't otherwise give. Go with your "first mind", if you think they want something from you, be prayerful that **you choose** to bless them, or give them what they want. Be aware that you are not taken advantage of; but go ahead, and enjoy your meal!

On a scarier note, in some cultures, food and beverage is used as the vehicle for pagan curses. But the Greater One is in you! Still consider the source of your *food blessings,* and don't forget to ask God's grace over your meals. Remember not only to pray that your food is physically safe to eat, but now you know to ask that it is spiritually safe to consume, as well.

Affirmations:
I bind whoredoms, sex sins, lusts and perversions,
Especially sins brought on by food;

I cast them out in the name of Jesus.
I loose the Holy Spirit, holiness and
Temperance in my life.
I am aware, alert and ask God for spiritual discernment so I am not deceived by anything.
Food is not entertainment.

(highly recommended: "Beware of Their Leaven", (Warning: "Believer Discretion Advised"), 3-tape audio or video, by Pastor Dwayne N. Hunt.)

A Hill of Beans

*E*sau traded his birthright for a hill of beans, I mean bean soup. He was so hungry, he swapped his blessings for food, (Gen. 25:30-33). Jacob fed his brother, Esau, then led him down the path of deception. You'd never do that, would you? It's never been done to you, has it? You would never trade your birthright of salvation and eternal life, for food, drink, good times, or fleshly desires, would you? You wouldn't be willing to trade eternal salvation for eternal hell, so you can party, and do what you want, while on this temporary flesh journey through earth? Would you?

That's what the devil wants to know. That's what the devil keeps asking, every time he offers you something. Will you trade your God-stuff, your gifts, your salvation, your promises and blessings for *food*? Is food all it takes? The devil will get that for you. Or will you trade it for sex; how about perverted sex? Does it take that, because he can get that for you, too. Will you trade it for murder? What is it for which you will trade your salvation, and your reward? Will you trade it for money, or fame? *What do you want?*

There are no promises or warnings about the consequences of what you want. The devil doesn't care about you, even though you may think he's getting you something to make you *happy.* He's a corrupt business man, who's saying, "*What do you want? What will you accept in trade to give me the thing(s) I want from you?"* Deceptively, the devil looks like he's in the business to get something *for you,* but he's really trying to *take something from you.* Satan would steal your soul, (mind, intellect, and emotions), but he can't, (if you're saved). The only way he can get it, is if you give it willingly, or its taken legally. Trading is legal. Deception is legal. If you accept something from the devil, then you have give up what you promised him. The devil wants you to trade your God-stuff for whatever he's offering. And with that trade, barter, or ***theft***, comes pain, torture, and torment — either now, or later — in hell..

> **The devil's ultimate goal is to affect your soul's eternal address; he wants you in hell with him.**

The purpose of the Jesus' wilderness temptation was to show the reality, and the gravity of the temptations that man may face, and model the proper response. Jesus had just gotten all of His credentials; He had just received the highest anointing: the Christ anointing. He was graced with full power, yet no man knew it yet. (The devil comes early and often.) Satan came offering worldly *gifts;* things to try to trade Jesus for what God had just given Him. What is the first thing the devil thought could tempt Jesus? Food.

The devil doesn't care, he will come for your gifts *before* they are even used, as he tried with Jesus. Many times, he comes before the gifts are received, or known about. This is why it is so crucial for children and teens to be taught, trained, and nurtured spiritually. Their lives need to be spoken in to, so they know who they are, and what their gifts and talents are, at the earliest age possible.

Let's Make A Deal was a game where people traded what they had, what they thought they had, or what they thought they were going to get, for things seen, and unseen. That's what the devil wants you to do, like Esau, when he was hungry, *make a deal.* And that's what worldliness is all about — to distract, tempt, and take away the gifts of God *before* they are used, or even realized. The devil may even make people aware that they have certain gifts; put a false value on them, then en-slave them for his purposes. For example, people may take certain God-given gifts, and pervert them for per-sonal financial gain. If the gifted person is made aware of their godly gifts, educated, trained, taught, is in proper relationship with God, and in proper fellowship with the saints, then they won't trade, or be tricked out of price-less God-gifts. Not to mention the prayer covering they'd be under because of being under authority, and in right relationship. If Esau had fully realized what his birthright was, he probably would not have traded it for food. And if you recall the story, Esau was out in the wilderness, alone, hunting. He was not in fellowship, but Jacob was connected to the family —. Take a lesson, here.

You Don't Have Anything To Lose

The, *"You don't have anything to lose",* lie has surely been presented to you. *"Go ahead, try it, do it, you don't have anything to lose".* You may not look like you have anything to lose; you may not even feel that you have anything to live for. You may not feel special, or set aside, or even know your purpose yet, but if God made you, you've got something of great value. And if the devil is pursuing you, that confirms it — you are, and have tremendous value. But what you have is not of value unless you:

- **Know** what you have,
- **Know** that it has value, and
- **Know** how to use it.

When someone asks you, *"What do you have to lose,"* you need to **know** that you have great gifts and abundance from God. But He didn't give it to you to lose it. Usually, the person asking the question is in the world, and can't recognize the God-things about you anyway. Don't take advice, counsel, or direction from the ungodly, (Ps. 1.1). **You have a lot, but it's not to lose, and it's not *for* losing —it's for winning!**

<u>Affirmations:</u>

My Salvation is more important to me than
anything anyone could offer me,
especially the devil.
I refuse and reject temptations, whether it is simply
food, or other obvious violations against God's
commandments.
My Soul's eternal address is with God, and my
soul will arrive safely, intact,
and to the glory of God.
God has given me many gifts, talents, and abilities.
I do not have anything that I am willing to lose.
I am victorious in Christ.
I am not made for losing.

(highly recommended: **The Three Anointings,** *by Pastor Dwayne Hunt, book and/or single audio, or video tape)*

Fattened Up For the Kill
(Sacrifice)

Hansel and Gretel, of storybook fame, wandered into hostile witch territory. The witch, cannibalistic, and slight of sight, perceived by their bony wrists that they were not fat enough to eat. So she set out to fatten them up. That is exactly what we do to the Thanksgiving goose, and then sing songs about it. The *fatted* calf was prepared for the once-prodigal son, (Luke 15:23). The fattened turkey looks better on the platter, and is considered to taste better. Bigger is better, it's the American way. Americans really like **fat**; *the very thing that was set aside for God.*

The witch offered Hansel and Gretel, everything they liked; and they ate. There would have been no strategy to offering them things they wouldn't eat. **Devilish temptations are always things you like**. To entice a person into a sex sin, the devil will send someone attractive. To entice an eating sin, that food that you really enjoy, will be made available to you — especially if you have declared a fast!

When fattened up, the witch was ready to consume

them. Just like the witch, after being baited with the things you desire, the devil begins the *switch*, or tries to spring the trap. Satan offers things you like for a reason, and it's not because he likes you.

Or the devil, even if he has access to you, because of, and in spite of your lifestyle and choices, may leave you alone, allowing you to feel secure, and comfortable, *for a while*. You may begin to think that your success is because of your own hard work. You may *be* working hard, but as long as you're not worshiping, and serving God, the devil may sit back, and let you think you're living the perfect life, (for a time). Satan won't offer many obstacles, (if any), if you're not serving God. If he did, then you might become distraught, and seek God. Now why would the devil want you to do that? If you're not saved, and serving God, you're going to hell anyway; the devil can spend his energy trying to wreck havoc on the lives of other people.

When you're comfortable, you'll be thinking, *"That can't happen to me, or I've got it made, or, I can do whatever I want, and there is no consequence".* That's the physical and mental comfort the devil wants you to trust in. *Watch Out!* Maybe you're also thinking:

- *"I don't need to go to church,*
- *I don't need to live in holiness, as long as I do my sin-*

ning out of town, where no one knows me.

- *If I'm selective with whom I sin, they won't tell, and I won't tell — it'll be okay.*
- *I don't need to read the Bible. I don't need to fast or pray, that's for sinners, heathens, and poor people!"*

The bait has been offered and taken, but the devil may be doing nothing right now, but watching you sink deeper, and deeper in sin. Sin without immediate consequence, makes the sinner believe falsely, that there are *no consequences.* Now that you're deceived into being *spiritually comfortable,* you believe that you don't need to change anything about yourself; you're perfect, and you've got life figured out. The reality is, you've done so much wrong stuff, but nothing has happened — so you think nothing is going to happen. You are fat in your *Comforts.*

Listen closely, do you hear the devil singing a song about a fat goose? It's fat now, it'll look much nicer on the platter; now that it's fat, it will embarrass God more. Just when you don't think anything is going to happen, that's when the devil tries to reel in the goose he's caught. You!

Fatter is more attractive, better tasting, better looking to the predator. Who might want **you** fat, in your spiritual comforts, your natural abundance, or even physically fat? Who's after you? The devil. Who might want you heavier than you should be, slower moving, weaker, not toned, out of condition — not able to run, physically, or *spiritually*? The devil, wants you fattened up for the kill.

A lot of Pentecostals say they are *running for their lives;* they mean physical running. By running, I believe God means to *work,* as a machine works. When a car motor *runs*, it is doing the thing it's supposed to do. You are supposed to run your course to the finish, (Acts 20:24). Running means doing what you're made, called, and anointed to do.

Thinking of marathon runners, thank God, we don't have to physically run *from* the devil, and it's a good thing, because how many *could*?

Spiritual fitness, (spiritual prosperity), means your prayers are instant, and without ceasing. You are thankful to God; you study the Bible, you Praise and Worship. You're also faithful in church, paying your tithes, and giving offerings. Your spiritual machinery is working, and ready to use, at a moment's notice. Your gifts are stirred up, you're in the full armor of God, and you're ready with Spiritual Warfare, if necessary — ***that's running.***

Consumed In Fat

*T*he Bible talks about being *consumed in one's fat.*

Not like the dagger stuck in Eglon, but God says that when we have success, prosperity and abundance; we get **fat** in our comforts, and forget Him. That's what He calls, *consumed in our fat.* God hates it when we are consumed in our own life, goals, and successes, to His exclusion, and what He has called us to do. God says we turn away from Him, when we get *fat.*

Remember when you didn't have a car, weren't you in great, (or better) physical shape then? Now that you have creature comforts, such as your house, your job, and a nice vehicle, don't those luxuries make you a bit more full around the waist? It's human nature to forget *what got you there.* That's the nature that God is talking about, when we get comfortable. Even physically, when you were on your way up, you exercised and took care of yourself. Now that you have the nice position at the office, the gym is not even on your schedule. What have you taken off your *spiritual schedule* now that you think you don't have to ask God to bless your efforts any more?

Being consumed in fat doesn't mean that heavy people don't serve God; some all the more. I'm not saying that rich people don't serve God. The *Comfortable* people are those who are **not** serving God, but they *think* they have everything they *think* they want. Those people believe that God is for the needy, or the poor; they may believe that God is for *who*, and *where they used to be*. But every heavy person isn't *comfortable* anymore than every thin person is. The temptation is when everything is going fine in life, to put God on a back burner, or in a cabinet for storage, in the fridge or freezer, to keep for later usage. If you have a problem or a need, you can call on God, but He can't be put on hold. Why? **Because God is the one who is really doing the calling, and when the person who is calling hangs up, the line goes dead.** By Mercy and Grace, He allows time for repentance and correction, but it will not always be this way.

But Jeshurun waxed fat, and kicked: thou art waxen fat, thou art grown thick, thou art covered with fatness; then he forsook God which made him, and lightly esteemed the Rock of his salvation. (Deut 32:15)

If you only *lightly esteem* God, He will lightly esteem you. Whether you are in your *Comforts*, or not, the way you treat God will be returned to you. Don't you have relatives who only call, or knock on your door when they want something? Do you think God is happy to see you *only when you have a problem?* Where is His Praise, Worship, and service when things are well with you?

When you're sending up a prayer, God may look down and see, it's only you. He sees the trouble you're in, He understands, He has compassion, but you're the one who comes to church sometimes, the one who pays the tithe sometimes, and never gives offerings. You're the one who remains silent, and seated during Praise and Worship. Don't be offended, but if you've only lightly esteemed God, you may have offended Him! Repent and rectify the problem, now!

You've got to Praise God, because when you open your mouth and Praise Him, you *highly esteem* Him. When you pay your tithes, and give offerings, you highly esteem God. When you study, and obey the Word, you highly esteem God. When you witness, and minister to others, you highly esteem Him.

But if you're a silent saint, He may be thinking, *Oh, it's the one who lightly esteems Me. I'll get to their prayer, when I get to it. I will attend to the prayers of the Righteous man, and Faithful woman, first.* God has a responsibility to bless those in His Family first, just as you bless your own children first and foremost. God knows that if He blesses you every time you have a problem, and you're not serving Him, that you will never truly serve Him. Even though you may say, *"God if you bless me this time, if you get me out of this, I promise to come to church regularly, I promise to tithe, I promise this, and I promise that..."* God knows you won't. How does He know? Because you haven't. He's gotten you out of stuff before, hasn't He? You've been seeing Him as a spiritual vending machine. You don't praise or worship, or give offerings to a vending machine; you only go to it when you want something out of it. You must not lightly esteem God. Develop relationship with Him; He's a friend that sticks closer than a brother, (Prov 18:24).

<u>Affirmations:</u>
I esteem God, the Rock of my Salvation;
I Praise Him!
I repent of ever lightly esteeming God,
and I purpose to serve Him with my whole self,
whether times are fat and Comfortable, or not.
I will not become Fat in Comforts,
but I will Remember the Lord God,
who gives me power to get wealth.
As the Lord prospers me Spiritually,
I will not fail to Serve, Worship, Praise, Attend
Church, Pray, Study, Share with others,
minister, and be a blessing.
I endeavor to be Spiritually Fit, not spiritually fat.
I will Highly Esteem, the Rock of My Salvation
I *Will* Praise the Lord.

(highly recommended: "Praise Positions", single audio or video tape by Pastor Dwayne Hunt.)

Spiritually Fat

Spiritually Fat does not describe a physical size. There are all kinds of *Spiritually Fat* people, and they are of all sizes. It describes several kinds of people. First, those who sit on the church pews, not only every Sunday, but also *every* service. They are there, because they are *supposed* to be. These Spiritually Fat are not holding the pew down, they are not bearing the Spirit up, necessarily; they are just there.

They are the kind of people who believe that the first person who applies for a job should get it. They think the ideal person for a position at an office, is the *one who came first.* They mistakenly believe that the employer is looking for a warm-body to fill the position. God has no responsibility to bless you because you are physically at church—anymore than you get the job, just because you came to the interview. You've got to bring your mind, experience, and skills to that job; and they need to match the needs of the employer. And you've got to bring your mind, body, and soul to church, and be there in spirit and in truth, (John 4:23). *Being* at church because of fear of God, fear of hell, fear of falling into

sin, is just a start. (God doesn't want a relationship simply based on fear). Some regulars are as *baby-
Christians,* who don't trust themselves out of the pastor's
sight. They are at church because they are *supposed* to
be there; not because of relationship with God. (Not yet;
but prayerfully, right relationship with God is growing.)

Some *baby-Christians* may have even been drawing
on the pastor's teachings, for years, or *decades.* They
soak up the Word, expressionless, or with great emotion,
waving hands, and excitement; shouting, *Amen!* These
appear to have their spiritual life together. But at the end
of worship, they put on *outside* faces, go back to work
and home, *business as usual.* Never a word, a prayer,
or any ministry flows through them. They collect the
Word for years, but do nothing with it; thereby staying
baby-Christians, (Heb 5:12).

God requires regular church attendance, (Heb 10:25).
In addition, reading Christian books, and listening to
study tapes, will enhance your knowledge of the Word.
But collecting all manner of godly, spiritual information
and never using it, is like putting an expensive, hand-
knit, cashmere sweater in a cedar chest and saving it for
a *special occasion.*

**Your life here on earth is a special occasion;
it's why you're here.**

The Word of God is for this special occasion, that's why God provided it. Most pastors don't preach heaven anymore; the Word you are hearing is for **now, it's for applying to your daily, real life**. Rhema is Living Word, and that is for right now.

If you don't know what to do with the Word, or how to use it, pray for wisdom and understanding. Ask for the Holy Spirit so you can rightly divide the Word, (2 Tim 2:15). Once you divide the Word, it's like eating, now you can take *bites* of it. You can take in as much as you need, when you need it — spiritual food, for spiritual fitness.

But if you know what to do with the Word, and you are among those who only harbor spiritual knowledge to use at church fellowships, that's another story. The choir already knows what you know. Why not take the Word out to your work place, your home, your community, and bless those who haven't heard the good news of the Gospel. Being miserly is a **FAT Demon**; it can make you *Spiritually Fat.*

Affirmations:
I receive and use spiritual food properly.
I reject spiritual fat.
I share and minister spiritual food to others as God leads. I reject a miserly spirit.

Fat In Revelation Knowledge

*P*raise God, you are past the place where you only *collect* spiritual information. Perhaps you have been witnessing, or ministering in the grocery stores, and highways and byways. You might even talk to people where you work, or at the bus stop. You may talk to people who may not be saved; Praise God! Maybe you are faithful in attending church, faithful in paying tithes, and giving offerings, faithful in studying the Bible, and faithful in ministry. Since God has been able to trust you with the little things in life, He may be now trusting you with revelation. God may be revealing new, and wonderful things to your heart, that you've never heard anywhere before. Things that set you on fire, or make your heart soar. What are you doing with it? If nothing, then you are Spiritually Fat on Revelation knowledge.

Perhaps you've written it all down in a book, a journal, or a manuscript. Do you have a collection of poems, short stories, or sermons that the Lord has given you; wisdom that the Lord may have even awakened you in the middle of the night to impart? Have you shared any of those things with anyone, *as God has led?* Perhaps you've been faithful to record the new melody you woke up singing, and perhaps He gave you the anointed words, as well. Is that song published, recorded, or even shared with the music ministry of your church? That song could heal, deliver, or uplift someone. You may not know who, but God knows. Revelation Fat is a terrible thing.

Are you wondering why your ministry isn't taking off? God's not holding you back; you are. Minister what God has already given you. Like Samuel, to Eli ministry often begins with service to another ministry, *first*. Be faithful to your church, and leaders, then God can bless you.

Thank God, you are talking to others, and it's great to share of what you've received, from man, *and* from God through revelation. If you are not receiving yet, keep the faith. When you speak to, or witness to someone out of your *own* relationship with God, you are much more effective than just repeating what the pastor said on Sunday. What the pastor said, was for *you*! Some of it may be for that sinner you're witnessing to, but God gives fresh manna from heaven, for each occasion. Share, don't covet revelation! The *miserly, covetous spirit* that won't share revelation is a **FAT Demon.**

A saved friend loves to call to talk about the Word. We'd share the Lord's bright light being turned on in our hearts, and minds; even though neither of us had a pulpit. We shared by telephone, e mail, cards, letters and notes — by any means that we could. We shared with others, even if it was only one person at a time, we *ministered* the good news of Jesus, and the revelation we

received by the Holy Spirit. And you can do that too.
That is ministry.

There are some spiritually fat who receive revelation
and keep it hidden. I'm not talking about Mary who
couldn't disclose information about the conception of Jesus; neither am I talking about information that the Lord
has instructed you *not* to share yet. Many times He gave
the prophet a word, and told him, *"Not yet."* John the Divine ate the words read from *the little book,* (Rev 10:9),
because it was not the time to share it yet. I'm talking
about sharing a word in season — and you know in your
Knower, it's a word in season. Your heart may be pound-
ing, your pulse may be racing, you're so excited, but fear
may have gripped you. Fear will cause you to sit on that
pew, when God is saying, *"Get up!"* Fear can make you
Spiritually Fat; *the spirit of fear* is a **FAT Demon.**

Affirmations:
I receive and use spiritual food properly.
I reject Spiritual Fat. I receive and share
revelation as the Lord directs; I do not harbor it.
I bind up, and cast out the spirit of fear in my life,
and I loose the spirit of Love,
Power and a Sound Mind, in the name of Jesus.

Fat In Gifts & Talents

*T*here are many who are *fat* in gifts and talents—I call it Gift Fat, or Talent Fat. Some can sing like a songbird, play an instrument, or build a bookshelf, masterfully, but they still sit on the pew. You've been a member of your church for five years, you've been to fellowship, after fellowship; you have God-given abilities, talents and skills but no one knows. That is also Spiritual Fat. Is it fear, or selfishness that keeps you seated, and keeps you from sharing? You've got yours, your salvation, your spiritual gifts, your house and car; do you care about anybody else?

Bob *majored* in photography in college, but worked in another field. No one in his church knew. The church's video minister moved out of state suddenly, but Bob told no one of his video-photography skills, because he didn't want to have to *"come to church all day, and tape."* The *spirit of selfishness* is a **FAT Demon**; it can lead to spiritual fatness. You will not be spiritually fit until you do what God says do. Be obedient.

<u>Affirmations:</u>
I receive and use spiritual food properly.
I reject spiritual fat.
I share willingly and gladly of my gifts
and talents that the Lord has given —

to the glory of God.
I reject selfishness, and self-centered-ness.
I reject Spiritual Fat of any kind in the
name of Jesus.

*(highly recommended: **"Accessing Divine Wisdom"**,
by Pastor Dwayne Hunt. Available on audio or video)*

Physically Fat

We have discussed several kinds of Spiritual Fat, which is the collection of spiritual, Bible-based information from any, and all sources, (especially from your pastor). We've discussed Revelation Fat, Talent Fat, and Gift Fat. You have a spiritual gift, and may even know what it is, but you don't move in it. That is not pleasing God.

And now for the meat of this book, (no pun intended), the physically fat, due to *spiritual causes*. People can be influenced by spiritual entities that drive them to **eat**. Every spiritual disorder that can lead to spiritual fat, can also lead to physical fat.

> **The things that are seen are brought to manifestation by the things which are unseen.**

The Bible tells us that the world we see is made by things which are unseen; the natural world that we see, reflects the spiritual world that we don't see, (Heb 11:3) The food on your plate is not the only thing *contributing* to your size. When you become spiritually fat, which is invisible; then physical, visible fat can follow. What unseen things may be affecting you, and your weight?

Candace left a church where she was flowing in ministry every Sunday, and teaching a weekly Bible class, for a church where she sits on the pew. She is collecting spiritually, but not *giving* spiritually; that leads to *Spiritual Fat*. What is spiritual has translated into the physical; Candace has gained 20 pounds (3 dress sizes) in just a few months.

This is not a fat-person bashing book; but it is a fat-bashing book. Anyone who is fat, didn't just become fat overnight. Chances are something happened that changed either eating patterns, physical activity levels and patterns, or both. Those changes may have influenced metabolic rates, (the way your body uses food), permanently, or temporarily. That something that happened may have been *spiritual, or had spiritual or soulish consequences.* You haven't stopped eating since so and so died. You never used to eat this much (or often) since the divorce. Your appetite picked up that summer you spent with relatives — now you eat as much as Little Cousin Junior. Soulish and spiritual things, though unseen, affect physical things that are seen — even your weight and size.

Most people don't want to be fat, (though some say

they do). Kids proudly stick out six-year old stomachs after a big meal. But by the time they are pre-teen, most want to be slim to prepare to participate in the activities of teenage, and early adult years. Who wants you fat? God? No. The devil? Probably; the devil personified by Hansel and Gretel's witch. Let's weigh things out — no pun intended. If you're physically running for your life, fat (fatter) can mean: slower moving, and easier to catch. If the devil is shooting fiery darts at us, (Eph 6:16), then our bodies must be targets. If a person is fat, then the target is easier to see, *and hit.*

If you are *spiritually* running for your life, then you are slower moving, and easier to catch; you don't feel like praising or worshiping, you don't feel like praying, you're too tired to read the scriptures, or go to Bible Study. And don't even think about asking you to serve as an usher, or in a church ministry! In that condition, if the devil threw a spiritual problem at you, you'd fall apart. Physically, or spiritually, you're at a disadvantage. You have got to make some changes!

Physical Changes

*M*uscles appear on the guy that works out, the opposite will happen to the Couch Potato. Muscles will disappear on the person that doesn't exercise. Muscles burn

the most energy in a body. If you don't have any muscles, you don't need as much food, no matter how **BIG**
you are. But folks with muscle can eat and eat, but don't
gain weight. And they **need** to eat, because that muscle
is using up energy and burning calories. Eating will not
make muscles, only making muscles, and using muscles
will make muscles. (I'm not necessarily talking about the
bulky body-builder type — just well-toned muscles.)

On the outside and the inside, God has designed a
remarkable body; it will change to reflect what you're doing with it. More aptly put, your body will reflect what
you're doing to it.

> ## Your Body Will Change To
> ## Reflect Your Lifestyle.

Spiritual *muscles* are also made by **use**. If you aren't
using any spiritual energy, you don't need to receive any.
This is how people dry up, spiritually — they are not giving out anything to anyone else, they are not ministering
what they've been given, to anyone else. They may get
fat for a while as they receive and receive spiritual food,
but soon, God will cut that off, and they will dry up, spiritually. This also happens physically; as long as you are
using muscles, they will prosper and be healthy, but
when you don't, fat adds on. After the fat, the muscles

atrophy; they become weak, and saggy, from neglect and not using them.

Physiologic Changes

Eat enough chocolate, sweets (cakes and bread), and drink enough alcohol, the body (flesh), will start to *crave* it. Remember when you hardly liked cola, and now you drink it every day. Certain changes happen in the body to make you *handle* it. Some people drink a beer and get *high* off of it, but a single beer the next time won't have the same effect. The body creates special cells that use up the alcohol, so more alcohol is needed the next time to have the same effect. The same thing happens with caffeine, and sugar in cola and chocolate, (not as obvious as with drugs and alcohol, at first.) This is how addictions begin.

Your body has certain cells that enjoy the sugar, and the alcohol, etc. As you eat more and more of the junk, the *"I-like-junk"*-cells grow in numbers. Now there are twice, or four times as many *junk-cells*; and they want to eat. They want you to feed them. They get more sugar in breads, cakes and alcohol, by creating a natural, or flesh **craving** in you. Feeding this craving creates the overgrowth, which creates the craving, which creates the overgrowths. It's a vicious cycle. The more junk-cells, the stronger the craving is. It's a very real need to you; it will wake you up at night. It will keep you from sleeping, unless you give into it, then it may calm down enough to let you go back to sleep. It will distract you at work; cravings and addictions have no clocks. They don't care where you are, or what you're doing, their job is to drive you to give in to what they want you to do. **It's real, it's spiritual; but it's not of God.**

Over-indulging in sugars, breads, and alcohol (for example), leads to an overgrowth of yeast in the body. This overgrowth of yeast causes chronic tiredness, mental dullness, dark circles around the eyes, and may contribute to allergies, and other problems. If in great numbers, those bad cells may overrun normal, healthy cells in the body, causing physical sickness. Yeast infections (overgrowths), are not always the kind they advertise the one or three-day cures for on television; and they don't just affect women. Also irregular eating can cause blood sugar surges, among other things. Too much of any thing is a big problem.

Affirmations:
I receive and use natural food properly;
I reject unhealthy fat.
I choose what I eat — it is not chosen for me.
Fat does not just happen.
My body burns calories and fat efficiently.

I am not willing to Lose anything else, but I am willing to Get Rid of Weights and Burdens In the Natural and Spiritual.

*(A good book to read is **The Yeast Syndrome** by Dr. John Parks Trowbridge, and Morton Walker, DPM).*

<u>Disclaimers</u>: *If you don't exhibit any eating, snacking, or dining excesses, that doesn't mean you don't have any spiritual concerns; this book is mainly about the causes of overeating, and the consequences of it, including fat. Do not mis-interpret* <u>The FAT Demons</u>, *to believe that God is giving you a clean bill of spiritual health if you don't find yourself in any of the preceding, or following categories.*

This book is not suggesting that everyone has a problem; it outlines some problems that may be caused by spiritual entities. Use Wisdom and the Holy Spirit to guide, and confirm any spiritual diagnoses and remedies. Medically, this book does not diagnose any physical ailments of metabolism, or other function. This book does not diagnose any emotional, psychological, or mental ailments. See your physician where indicated. This is a spiritual reference.

The
FAT Demons

There are some spirits that influence and promote bad habits such as, drinking, smoking, and drug abuse. And there are spirits that influence **eating**; I call them **FAT Demons**. They are sent to encourage overeating, eating the wrong foods, eating to distraction, or obesity; to the end of not only not serving God, but by omission, or lifestyle, serving the devil. If eating is, or can be a temptation to you, then food is what the devil will use to tempt. If you're a Jack Sprat, (who could eat no fat), then the devil won't offer you food. But Jack had a wife who would *eat no lean;* that's who will be tempted by food and snacks.

People need deliverance from the spiritual oppression of putting things in their mouths, such as drugs, alcohol, and *food.* Babies and children try everything in their mouth. You have probably been told, *"Don't put that in your mouth",* more times than you've been told anything else in your entire life. If you are still being told that about spiritual things, then you have not graduated from being a baby-Christian. *Don't put that in your mouth,* or *take that out of your mouth*, is a parent's mantra. There must be a reason God wanted you to hear those words so often. Putting wrong things in the mouth is a temptation for too many, *Christians included.*

You have probably been told,
Don't put that in your mouth, or take that out of
your mouth, more times than
you've been told anything else in your entire life.

Food addiction is a reality. The demons' (fallen angels), assignments are predictable. They are seeking to destroy God's work in the earth, with tested and tried spiritual weapons. You are not the first person to be tempted by food, excess, or sin. The assigned demon knows what you like, and how to present it to you. A demon will not offer pork chops to Jack Sprat; **where there is no desire, there is no temptation.** The demon's charge is to present something that will tempt, to bring disgrace to you, and God's kingdom, if possible. We pray that it isn't.

Have you ever had the feeling that someone doesn't like you? You're right. The devil hates you, and is working *against* you. Let me give you an idea of how much the devil hates you — add up all the hateful, spiteful, hurtful things *all* the people you have known in your life have done to you. Satan hates you **more** than all of that hate added together, because he put all of those people up to doing those things against you, and is *still* working against you. Satan puts what's taboo in your path, and within your grasp, then tries to influence you to take it. If you're a thief, the opportunity to steal something you really want to steal will present itself. If you're an alcoholic, or drug user, he'll make those things available to you. If you are a food-aholic, ***then dinner's served.*** For Adam & Eve, it was forbidden fruit; what is it for you? What is your weakness? You don't have any; the devil can't get you that easily, *you think*?

The devil will start with something that seems harmless, then try to move you to the sin where he really wants you. The *spirit of lust*, for example begins with vanity. Oh, there's nothing wrong with caring about your appearance. But the *spirit of vanity* comes in, and is nurtured when you cater to it, by spending way too much time, money, and putting too much importance on how you look. Then vanity makes room for lust; *don't you want others to notice how lovely you are? That's how it starts.*

You've got to be spiritually alert at all times

Other spiritual oppressions can start with *food. The devil's got food for bait; like a mouse trap, and you're the mouse.* He's got things you like, hoping to open the door for other distractions, dangers and sin. The devil is trying to get your soul. What bait are you susceptible to; what are you likely to put in your mouth? Watch out for devil hooks, and mouse traps, attached to that *cheese.*

Affirmations:
I bind, and cast out every Snack Demon, Dining
Demon, Eating Demon, every FAT Demon;
I bind up, and cast out the spirit of obesity
in the name of Jesus.
I loose the spirit of Health and Wellness.
*I will obey my Momma — finally
and take things out of my mouth
that don't belong there.*
I purpose to study to show myself approved, and
to be alert at all times of the strategy of the Enemy
so I can be victorious to the Glory of God.

*(highly recommended: **HSGD**, (Hunt's Spritual Gifts Discovery) a test booklet, and discovery of where you really belong in ministry. By Pastor Dwayne N. Hunt).*

Fat Mouths & Fat Prophecy

Girl, if you don't stop eating ..... you're going to be big as a house!" How many well-meaning relatives have spoken those words to you?

"He's big-boned, like his daddy, he's going to be the size of a football player." How do you know?

How about these warnings: "You won't always be a size 8, just wait until you get a little older."

"Wait until your first baby, wait until you're 30; wait until you live a little longer, you'll see! Wait until gravity hits, the midriff bulge, the love handles... You've got big feet, you've got a big head, so the rest of you.... You eat like a horse,... You're going to be big as a cow..." Do I need to go on? **These are all words of the Fat Prophets.**

Who told them they could prophesy over you? Then why are you listening to them? Just because someone is older than you, doesn't make them your personal prophet. They have no authority to speak into you life — unless you allow it. Just because a Fat Prophet told you you'd be fat, (even if it was your *mother*), doesn't mean you have to be fat. Fat Prophets are just regular people, with a lot of opinions, and loose jaws. There are even examples of people doing similar things in the Bible. Do you remember the big deal about Ham looking on Noah's nakedness, and the resulting cursing of Canaan? God didn't do the cursing, (false prophecy), Noah did. As Ham is supposed to be the father of Canaan, the Black race is supposed to have been cursed to be servants ever since. **Not so.** God did not commission Noah to operate in the Prophet's office and curse the whole Black race, especially at that time: *Noah had a hangover!* (Genesis 9:21-25).

So who are these people who have been, and still telling you what size you are going to be? Fat Prophets. False Prophets.

There are countless thousands of people over 30 who still wear a size 8, and thousands of women who have had babies, who don't have pot-bellies, or love handles. There are thousands over 40, 50, and older, in a size 10, or whatever size *they choose.* You do not have to gain weight just because you had a birthday. When a child, is 5, he may wear a size 5, and a size 10 when 10; that's the way it is with kids. But lordy, you don't have to wear a size 40W just because you're 40. Ladies and Gentlemen: you have dominion over your body, you can be any size **you** choose to be! The Fat Prophets are False Prophets; they have lied, and do lie.

What are you going to do about all the lies that have been spoken over you all your life? As faith comes by hearing (Rom 10:17), you should be hearing what thus saith the Lord, instead of what thus saith Aunt Sally. She's told you how many times, what mac & cheese is going to do to your thighs? You've also heard that you're going to keep eating it. For one, regarding the mac & cheese, why are you still eating it? And, two, why are you letting it do that to your thighs? Instead of not eating it, or eating, then exercising, proving the Fat Prophets wrong? Are you trying to prove Aunt Sally right? Then you can say, *"My Aunt Sally is a prophet, she can tell who is going to be fat"*.

Fat Prophets are only speaking what they hear, what others have said over them, and what they may want to happen to you anyway. They can be right, you can be fat. Or they can be wrong; you get to choose by *your* actions. Don't let the Fat Prophet's words dictate to you. (And by the way, they've told you some other wrong stuff too, but this book is about fat). Let all that wrong stuff go; release it to God. Ask Him if it's true. As for these "prophets", they aren't being very spiritual; if they were, they'd be saying what God says about you, not just reporting what they <u>see</u> with their natural eyes.

Maybe It's You?

*H*uh? Are you your *own* Fat Prophet? Are you thinking fat thoughts about yourself? Are you racked with guilt about your weight? Are you increasing the weight of guilt you now carry by *saying* negative things about your weight, your size, your shape, or the way you look in, or out of clothes? What are you saying about your own desire, or lack of desire and discipline to exercise? Are you talking to yourself, and others about how fat you are? Then you are your own Fat Prophet; the *devil* has trained you well.

"If I just walk past the dessert cart, I'll gain weight." Now you know that's not true. Is it funny? No. Can you find something else to make fun of? *"If I smell food cooking, it puts on pounds."* Is that true? No. Is it funny? No. Stop prophesying fat over your body, and over yourself. You're operating the bad, man-made principle of: *Fat Comes by Hearing.*

God says that faith comes by hearing, (Rom 10:17); what I'm talking about, is **talking about Fat**. Keep your mouth shut with the Fat Jokes, and it will be easier to keep it shut when that forkful of sweet potato pie, (or cheesecake), comes dancing in front of your face.

You can be your *own* worst enemy, the world says. You can be your *own* Fat Prophet. Faith comes by hearing. How do you expect your body, size, and weight to *decrease,* if you keep talking it up. (Unless you're a liar, and *you* don't believe a word <u>you</u> say. Think about it.) Maybe you don't have anyone to blame it on, but you. You can change. Here's how:

- **Stop** making Fat Jokes about yourself, it's not making anybody like you more, *especially your body*.
- **Stop** saying what Fat is going to pile on if you eat, go near, or smell food. Are you a comedian, or a real person?
- **Stop** telling yourself how hungry you can get, and bragging about how much you can eat — a cow, a horse, an ox, etc. It's not funny; you're not in grade school anymore.
- **Stop** making fun of your shape, your size, and any body parts that you don't like.
- **Stop** *thinking* any of these things about yourself, in public, or private. (Cast down the thoughts before they become words, 2 Corinthians 10:5). If you don't know what to think on, try: Philippians 4:8.
- **Stop** squeezing yourself into things. Break free! Break free so you can move! Compressing fat keeps it fat. No one puts on a girdle to exercise.
At least if you're up and about, your walking can bene-

fit you somewhat. But if the muscles aren't moving, they won't be burning any calories, or fat. Break free!

Yes, I said girdle! If you're willing to be uncomfortable for hours at a time — try exercise! Don't wear your clothes so tight that you have discoloration, and bruises on your skin. You've got to make some changes when under wires, or hook closures are digging in, and marking your skin.

- **Stop** trying to please others. If your spouse likes you heavy, and you want to be slimmer and fitter; you're going to have to please yourself. (That's another whole book).
- Get to know yourself.
- Learn to like, and love yourself, In Christ.
- When feeling hungry, discern which are emotional (Soul Cravings) to you, what is a Flesh Cravings, and discipline yourself   accordingly. *(See* **Soul Cravings**, *page 87)*.

Don't be afraid to say, *"I desire to be healthy, and physically fit"*. (Whatever that is to you). Don't be afraid to **say** what you really want, even though it may sound funny the first time you hear yourself say it. Exercise your faith, then exercise your body! The Bible says we shall have whatsoever we say, (Mark 11:23). Don't be caught saying one thing at home, then making fun of yourself in public; that's double-mindedness, bordering on self-hatred. Your kids will think you're *loco*, then they'll copy that self-defeating, self-deprecating behavior. You can be healthy and physically fit — if that's for you, then claim it, speak it, then do what it takes to be it!

- **Stop** saying how you can't lose weight like you used to.

Metabolism doesn't necessarily have to decrease with age. Usually what changes is lifestyle, (diet), and activity levels. Remember that you have **dominion** over your body — which includes how it works, how it moves, how it serves you, and everything else it does. **Start telling your body what to do**, and how to do it. That's what the fat talk is doing. It's telling your body the *opposite* of what you really want.

Have the faith to say what you really want. Faith talk sounds like this: *"My body works efficiently, and I burn calories and fat the way God intended."* Or, *"I am healthy and physically fit."*

Don't give up; God is the Lord over all flesh, and that includes yours. And with God, all things are possible. The Word says not to be led by the flesh, that is not just talking about emotions and Soul Cravings; it's talking about Flesh Cravings too. Do not let cravings and *"I wants"* lead you. If you allow the Spirit to lead, you will walk in temperance, self-control, health and fitness.

**Come unto me, all ye that labour and are heavy laden,
and I will give you rest.
Take my yoke upon you, and learn of me; for I am
meek and lowly in heart: and ye shall find rest unto
your souls.
For my yoke is easy, and my burden is light.
(Matt 11:28,30)**

The Lord is inviting those who are **heavy laden** to come to Him. He will give rest (restoration), to your souls. He further says that His yoke is easy, and His burden is light. That tells us that the burden of the Enemy is **not easy**, it is difficult; nor is it light, instead it is heavy. That's how you'll know the difference between God's yoke, and the devil's burdens. All that stuff you're trying to carry around is the devil's; all those emotions, all that hurt, all that guilt, shame, and depression, is the devil's. All that physical weight, is a manifestation of the spiritual oppression; it is not of God, it is of the devil.

Come to Jesus and be restored to what God intends you to be. Getting saved doesn't mean all natural consequences of sin suddenly disappear, but if the sin never stops the consequences never stop either. If you're already saved, but *going through*, then be thankful that you have a relationship with Him that gives you the victory, and restores. Be thankful that you have the Holy

Spirit, and use Him as the Comforter.

As faith comes by hearing, it's time you start hearing some right things. From whom? Yourself, for starters. The **Affirmations** provided in this book are good as a beginning. Use them to be your own prophet. Be a Thin Prophet, a Slim Prophet, a Fit Prophet a Health Prophet, over yourself.

Faith for good things comes by hearing good things. Faith comes by hearing. How many people have *you* prophesied skinniness to? And aren't they skinny? Remember when you also couldn't gain an ounce, no matter how much you ate? Wasn't there a Slim Prophet pronouncing that over you? Maybe that Slim Prophet, was *you*. Remember when you used to look in the mirror, and tell yourself how good you looked? What changed? Why did you stop? Are you waiting for someone else to do it? The words you hear, were the first things that changed, the spirits that you allowed to influence you were the next things to change. Then your natural eating and exercise habits changed. Faith comes by hearing. Fat comes by hearing. Skinny comes by hearing. Guard your ears! Decide what you want to hear from now on, it will affect what you become!

Affirmations:
I reject all false prophecy, the words that any Fat

Prophet has spoken over me.
I can have what I say —therefore,
I rebuke myself if I have spoken Fat over my body.
I will exercise my Faith, and my body.
I Stop all negative talk and thinking toward myself,
and about myself.
I love myself, in Christ.
I love myself.
I choose what size I want to be,
it is not chosen for me.
I choose health and life!
I choose what I eat; it is not chosen for me.
I break free out of girdles and tight things, so I can
MOVE!
The devil is bound, and cast out, not me.
Excess weight is the devil's burden
I am anointed of God;
the devil's burden is destroyed
because of the anointing.
I am anointed, therefore I am free!

(highly recommended: **Behave,** *mini-book, by Dr. E. Marlene Hunt, and* **"Let It Go",** *by Dwayne Hunt, single audio or video).*

The Spirit of Obesity

Fat Prophets can speak the *spirit of obesity* into people's lives. The spirit of obesity is made up of the imps and entities that I call the **FAT Demons**, et. al. What do **FAT Demons** do, and what does **FAT Demons**-work look like?

People try and try to lose weight, but it doesn't seem to happen. There is a trend in families where everyone is heavy. When whole families live in the same house, and have the same diet and exercise patterns; yet there are big differences between sizes, we wonder what's behind what is seen. What is it that takes over a whole family for generations, or one member, causing fat? Could it be a spirit of obesity? Yes, **FAT Demons**, the same that the Fat Prophets minister with their words.

The *spirit of obesity* can be:

- Generational – runs in families to 3rd and 4th generations.
- Transferred – by contact, association, relationship, marriage
- Influencing – makes suggestions for the victim to follow .

- Oppressive – weighs down by sin, or bondage of sin.
- Possessive – resides with the person all the time.

The spirit of obesity, headed up by the *spirit of whore-doms,* may have a number of little demons under it, which I have given easy to understand names, such as the *Dining Demons, Snack Demons, Chocolate Demons, Eating Demons, Coffee Demons, Ice Cream Demons,* etc., whatever foods the devil may try to use to bring on obesity.

How do these demons influence, or possess? They can't unless *you, or someone you're related to* invites, or lets them into your life. When your child begs for a cookie, and you give in, that's the end of it. But a demon nags until you resist unequivocally, or give in. If you resist, that's not the end; that demon, (or another), will try again. If you give in, that's the beginning. The relentless nature of spiritual attack, puts you in a spiritual war zone. (You've always wanted to be popular, you are — you are spiritually popular, like it or not.) Because demonic spirits travel together, if one is allowed in, it invites it's *cousins*; which are like squatters looking for a place to dwell. The first demon who wants to visit or camp in your popular place (your body), may be a Dining Demon. You, and a lot of other Christians, may judge a Dining Demon socially, and spiritually acceptable. These demons are excused with, *"Oh, she just has a big appetite*. Or, *"You know, Bro. John, he's all man".* Or, *"Girl, you really know foods, you must be a gourmet".* These eating disorders are trivialized, or made fun of. But once the demon gets in, it beckons for its cousins, which may **not** be socially, or spiritually acceptable. It's cousins are Smokers, Drug Users, Alcoholics, Adulterers, Sex Perverts, Gamblers, and Murders, etc. But the only way they can get in, is if you invite them in.

Further, a demon cannot be appeased or satisfied. They don't make deals, they just come to do what they have been instructed to do. Demons don't compromise — you can't reason with a demon. When you give in, thinking, *I'll just do this just this one time*; you've just sprung the trap. The influencing, or possessing demon isn't leaving after you indulge once —that's only the beginning. That's why there are generational oppressions and possessions — *they don't leave* on their own. If they are not put out — kicked out — they stay. They just wait for folk to die, and then influence, oppress and possess their children into the same sin acts and bondages. A good man leaves an inheritance to his children's children. A spiritually cursed man does the same thing; only it's not good, it's demonic.

So when you think, *I'll just have one more, then I won't ever do that again.* Don't deceive yourself. It may not be very easy to get over a bad habit, or behavior; the influence of the demon may have graduated to an addiction, and or, a spiritual possession by that time. If you don't care much about yourself, think about your children, (born and unborn), before you make the spiritual decisions that you are faced with.

It's easiest never to give in to demonic influence. It's easiest never to start a bad habit. Depending on your spiritual predisposition, resisting may not be easy, but it is easier than getting over it. It's easier than suffering through it, it's easier than wasting time, money, and your life away, until deliverance. It's easiest for your children, never to pass it on to them. It may not be easy to resist, but it's the easiest of all possible scenarios.

Don't give in to the **FAT Demons!** They don't leave readily, especially if you feed them. That means don't give into their urgings, influence, and cravings. They don't die. If fed, they multiply. They try to increase in number, and then they try to cause you to increase in **size.** That is not the kind of multiplication you want! Resist the **FAT Demons!**

Affirmations:
I bind up, and cast out the spirit of obesity and any
work of the FAT Demons in my life,
and generationally in my family.
I block and renounce every association and

friendship that gives place to FAT Demons.
I loose the spirit of God, the spirit of health, wellness and Life, in the name of Jesus.

The Dining Demon

*Let's go out to dinner. Will you meet me for lunch?
Let's grab a pizza Saturday night.* A meal is always a good excuse for a date. Food is often the ice-breaker to start a new relationship; (good or bad). The *spirit of adultery,* and the *spirit of fornication*, both encourage eating. Their activities can center around eating, or the pretense of eating. Worldly specialists say if a mate's weight is mysteriously going up, (or down) watch for cheating. The person may be juggling another relation-ship, that may revolve around meals. Or they could be innocently losing or gaining weight. But sudden weight loss, (in a healthy individual), could be the result of the *spirit of vanity*, or it could invite *vanity.* As said before, *vanity* invites *lust.* See how these oppressions work to-gether?

The *adultery*, or *fornicating spirit* is not sneaking *food* on the side, it is sneaking sex; it is working *with* it's cousin, the Dining Demon, using food as the cover-up, (with horrible side-effects, and consequences). But it may have all started with a seemingly innocent dinner invitation. See how the devil uses something simple, and adds it to something bad, to cause something worse.

Food-wise, the Dining Demon has class. It knows what to order, it eats in good restaurants, it knows all the courses, such as the appetizer, soup du jour, entrée, etc. It knows the best cuts of steaks and prime rib; and this demon knows desserts. This spirit influences, or possesses by making folk believe they have *arrived* because of food and wine knowledge, style, etiquette, and the ability to *afford* the lifestyle that goes with it. This does not mean don't go out to dinner, but if you feel that you have overeaten, and overspent every time you dine out; if you feel guilty, or some other oppressive emotion, then there may be a spiritual component to this that you need to look in to.

Maybe you've been told that you have an eating disorder; perhaps you do. Perhaps you don't. The problem may just be an influencing spirit causing the symptoms of over eating. Maybe it's a Dining Demon causing your voracious appetite.

Conversely, the Holy Spirit, dwelling in you, will cause you to exhibit discipline, moderation, self-control, and temperance.

The Snack Demon, et. al
*T*he Snack Demon is more of a blue-collar, every-day

demon. It influences the sneaking of food, for eating in private. The Snack Demon has you hiding food in secret places. Eating in the *bathroom* is not off-limits for the Snack Demon. (Is that disgusting, or what?)

Have you ever noticed how most very heavy people aren't seen eating very much, but they maintain their weight? You've asked yourself, *when* are they eating? They sneak food when no one is looking. (I hope that's not a surprise to you.)

God says don't over eat, but the Snack Demon and Chocolate Demons, *(and others),* are sent to encourage, convince, influence, even possess the mind to do things against the express will of God. One such possession is evidenced in the story of the pigs that drowned. The pigs had received the 2000 demons that had been in *one* man; Legion. When the spirits entered the pigs they ran off a cliff, and drowned in the sea, (Mark 5:9-13). The demons wanted some living place to reside. When they were in the man, they made the man crazy; when they entered the pigs, then the pigs committed suicide. (Sueycide, *pun intended*).

These hellish demons have been sent as emissaries, of the devil, and they want to dwell in you. They lead folks into temptation and sin, so the devil can say to God, *"I told you so"*. Satan is an accuser of the brethren, and the *womenren*, and the children. *Even if he's only accusing you of food abuse, or overeating. (But he de-sires worse sins of you).*

Have you ever eaten, then wondered to yourself, *"Why did I eat that? I wasn't even hungry, or didn't even really want that."* We're not going to say the devil made you do it. Perhaps there are things in your life that are influencing you, subconsciously; that you may not have 100% control over your life, as you should. If you feel bad, guilty, (voices of the lying Fat Prophets, in your head don't count); weak, or oppressive feelings after eating, then suspect negative spiritual influence.

Eating for the sake of eating, not for nourishment, is a trick of the enemy. Advertisers make snacks look like entertainment. They want you to believe that movie plots are better if you're eating, ball games are more fun, etc. But none of that is true, or accurate. After indulging, there may be discomfort, or bloating. After the pounds pile on, misery, depression, feelings of being unattractive, among other emotions, may compound the issues. Who remembers or cares about the plot of the movie, or the score of the ball game after the problems from over-eating show up, namely fat, irregularities in metabolism, or disease?

Do you know why you set those snacks out in the first place? Habit? Do you have the habit of eating buttered popcorn when watching TV? Who told you that you wanted the food? No one, right. The Snack Demon. The Snack Demon is real, it's job may be to make you think you're hungry, not getting your share of food, or not satisfied. It's not cute, funny, nor is it something to brag about.

Check yourself: If you are hiding food, or carrying it around in your purse, (not for your children, or a medical condition), that may be a sign of food addiction, or over-eating; in response to the influence the *spirit of obesity's* Snack Demon. Food that is eaten in your car, and in places when no one is watching, is still food; it still has fat and calories. That which is done in darkness will surely be brought to light; especially sunlight, in that swimsuit at the beach.

Affirmations:
I bind, and cast out every Snack Demon, Dining Demon, Eating Demon, every FAT Demon; I bind, and cast out the spirit of gluttony and the spirit of obesity, in my life, in the name of Jesus. I loose the Holy Spirit and the spirit of wellness, Health, physical vitality and fitness I choose Life.

THE GOD OF HEALTH
Eating With The Enemy
By Minister Erma Simpson, *Basic Moves Ministry*

When you sit down to eat with a ruler, consider carefully what is before you; and put a knife to your throat if you are a man given to appetite. Do not desire his dainties, for they are deceitful foods.
(Prov. 23:1-3)

Hunger vs. Appetite:

Hunger is a God-given desire for man's physical survival. Hunger is triggered by biological need for food. (Most Americans have never experienced true hunger. The growling that we feel, is the stomach letting us know that it is empty, most times it is simply asking for water, not food.

Appetite is craving (Lust) triggered by the sight, taste, smell, or even thought of food. Appetite causes us to overindulge (gluttony) in food, and to desire foods that God has not recommended.

Note: Hunger may be satisfied while appetite persists. After a meal, no man is hungry when he reaches for dessert! Many times appetite rather than hunger causes us to desire, and eat foods that are not good for us.

Published with permission

Whoredoms

*W*horedoms, (worldliness), is a spirit. Under it's demonic umbrella is the lust for money, prostitution, adultery, fornication, idolatry, chronic dissatisfaction, excessive appetite, and other things. *Whoredoms* drives the lusts for the feelings and experiences of the flesh life, that lead to disaster, death, and eternal damnation.

Idolatry

*P*eople hear the word *whoredoms* and may think of Hosea and his harlot wife, Gomer. But they will not think it has anything to do with them. News Flash*: Whoredoms* includes those who love to eat, *idolaters*, and a lot of others.

When you say, *"I just love Michael Whomever, and he eats a certain breakfast cereal, so that's what I have to eat"*; that's idolatry. The world is filled with copy-cats; that's how most things are sold to people. Folks want to be like the "Mikes" of this world; and that's why celebrity endorsements work. Those stars and athletes may not even eat the food, or use the product they advertise! If you're copying the image presented in TV ads—that's idolatry.

Or you might say, *"I just love ice cream, I have to have it every day. I have to have my chocolate, or I gotta have my coffee"*. Perhaps you are saying these things to be conversational, mainstream, or clever. Do you really want to be identified by a *food*? Didn't your mama call you *Pumpkin* long enough? Wouldn't you rather be identified by the name of Jesus? Do you want people to say, *"There she is, run get her some coffee, before she snaps"*, or *"Look, there's a woman of God, I wonder if she has a word from the Lord today?"*

Try this, *"I just love God, I've gotta have God, every-day"*. Pant after God, crave God; worship God. We were not put here to worship food; that's idolatry. Some people say they love to eat, some live to eat. We should just eat to live. Amen.

Jesus tells us to have bread and wine in Remembrance of Him at Communion. That belongs to Jesus, and no other. Pagan religions pay homage to false gods, and to the dead, by preparing special meals, and pouring libations. If we are offering food and drink to any other than God, isn't that idolatry?

Affirmations:
I repent of not putting God first

in all things in my life.
I repent of worshiping, lusting after,
or seeking anything ungodly in my life.
I repent of not acknowledging God in my Life's
choices, even my daily life,
God cares about everything I do,
and everything I choose.
I vow to seek God to direct my steps from now on.
I bind up, and cast out the spirit of idolatry in the
name of Jesus.
I loose Temperance, Self-control and
Spiritual deliverance in the name of Jesus.

Excessive Appetite

Excessive appetite is caused by a spirit. God says that the man that is given to excessive appetite should take a knife to his own throat, (Prov. 23:2). Suicide is not God's way. Is He saying that chronic overeating is suicide? Maybe. Probably. *Excessive appetite* is a spiritual problem; for which deliverance is needed.

Relatives tried to avoid Ted's house on the way to the park, because he'd eat their picnic lunches. He just ate and ate. Ted didn't inquire when people walked by with picnic baskets, or merely accept when offered food. Ted asked people sitting in his house, *"Did you pack a lunch?*

What did you bring?" Insisting, he would cause car trunks to be unlocked, and picnics foraged. If he saw food, he ate it. Sadly, he died a young man, at about 350 pounds. *Excessive appetite*, is a **FAT Demon**, and can be a killer demon.

Eat Like A Bird

*S*ome people believe they are hungry about every two hours; so they feed that hunger drive. Metabolically, it could be so, (hypoglycemia). People who are hungry every two hours usually *eat like birds*. Birds eat a lot; they eat little bits, often. That is actually good for you. The little bits are fruits, nuts, vegetables, and healthy foods that are quickly metabolized. These people are usually as thin as rails.

But many adults who take two hour *feedings*, are fat. They may have somehow confused the feeling of full, with the confession of empty; and set out to *refill* their stomachs. The full stomach may have been learned in childhood, but it is not optimum for good health.

But I'm Still Hungry!

Yes you are. With the deluge of processed foods on the market today, and the depletion of basic soil supplements in much of the farm land that grows the real vegetables we have to select from, many foods are lacking the very vitamins and minerals they are supposed to have. Even if you eat balanced meals, you may find yourself feeling as though you've missed something in your diet. Chances are, that you something was missing from your food. But eating more of the food may be too much food for your body. If you are one who experiences this, look into getting a vitamin supplement to supply your body with the essential substances it needs, but continue to eat as balanced meals as possible, while limiting the processed foods as much as you can. Don't overstuff yourself because of low nutritional value in the foods from which we must choose.

The stomach is not supposed to feel full all the time.

Chronic Dissatisfaction

*H*ow often have you craved something, but couldn't exactly put your finger on what that something was? A dill pickle could have been the beginning of an eating bonanza, then a banana split, followed by a pizza. You may have sent your spouse out late that night, for a burrito to top it all off. The next morning you realized that none of those things hit the spot, so you kept eating interesting things. A three-day-eating-binge later, you finally admit that the flavor experience, or sensation you sought never came in contact with your taste buds.

Some of the dishes you ate came close, but they weren't made quite right, too much salt, not enough garlic, wrong sauce; nothing really *satisfied.* But you ate so much of so many strange things, that you got tired of eating, or started to feel guilty about over-eating, and simply stopped the binge, but did *not* get **satisfaction.**

Did you **pray** while in binge-mode? What? Pray about food? Yes, you do it all the time. You do it every time you sit down to a meal. (Don't you?) You pray that the food will be safe to eat, nourishing to your body, some pray that it will taste good. *Why not also pray that the food will be satisfying to you?*

> And the LORD shall guide thee continually,
> and satisfy thy soul in drought, and make fat thy bones:
> and thou shalt be like a watered garden, and like a
> spring of water, whose waters fail not. (Isa 58:11)

The world may suffer of chronic dissatisfaction, it is spiritual, and a part of *whoredoms.* The Rolling Stones sang *"I Can't Get No Satisfaction"* in the 1960's, but the very wise Solomon wrote about satisfaction first, even *before Christ.*

**All the labour of man is for his mouth, and yet
the appetite is not filled. (Eccl 6:7).**

Man is ever working to fill his appetite, whether for
food, or material goods; yet Solomon says it is never satisfied. The Israelites were never sated in their appetites;
they were unhappy about the lack of water, and food.
They weren't pleased about the manna, they didn't like
the wilderness; they liked slavery better. They complained about snakes. With all that livestock they had
with them; we don't even know what they said about the
flies! Would you have complained? How many of you
would have told God that you couldn't leave Egypt because of all the **bugs** in the wilderness? Don't answer
that.

Sin Cannot Satisfy

*A*s wise and rich as King Solomon was, he wasn't
satisfied. He acquired 700 wives. Those wives practiced
idolatry and strange religions; which was the cause of
Solomon's downfall. As debase as the lifestyles were in
Sodom and Gomorrah, they still weren't satisfied. The
men wanted to have sex with the *angels* God sent.
Why? Because **sin cannot satisfy**. That's why you
can't commit a sin, and be done with it. It will leave you
unsatisfied, or dissatisfied. There was an old R & B

song, *"Do It 'Til You're Satisfied, whatever it is, do it..."*
That can't happen, since sin cannot satisfy. Worldly
songs are always asking for one night with a certain person who is the object of another's desire. If not one
night, the singer will ask for one illicit kiss, or something
else that seems almost innocent; thinking that one will be
enough for them. But it's not! If you were to get that one
opportunity, and act on your desire, you'll be thinking on
it, wondering about it, or maybe wishing, or planning to
do it another time — *just to get it out of your system.* **Doing it, is what gets it into your system!**

No matter how perverse, exotic, exciting, or whatever
you want to call it; no matter how frequently you do it —
sin cannot satisfy. This is why a sinner falls into bondage; repeating the sin act over and over. Man may
choose different partners, different settings, even different substances, but he can never get satisfaction from
sin. There is not enough *food* to satisfy, there are not
enough *drugs*, there is not enough *sex*.

> **Sin cannot satisfy — only God can satisfy.**

I am saved, and in the Body of Christ, I expect **Satisfaction**. God has promised it to me. If there is a *spirit of
chronic dissatisfaction*, then there must be a ***Spirit of***

Satisfaction; that spirit that fills you when you get blessed by God. Every blessing from God, small or large should be accompanied by this feeling. It's that *Spirit of Satisfaction* that I want everyday. I want it, I ask for it, I receive it, in the name of Jesus.

I want my children to have the *spirit of Satisfaction*, so they don't ask me to buy so many things in the stores. So they don't want to eat every time they see someone else with food. So they don't throw down the toy they have in their hand, and cry for their little playmate's toys.

I will abundantly bless her provision:
I will satisfy her poor with bread. (Ps 132:15)

Know the difference between satisfaction and complacency. Be, and strive for the best — for excellence. Students should not be satisfied with a D, when they can earn an A or a B. The normal child who is happy with the D, is complacent. God has promised us exceeding, abundantly, above what we ever expect, (Eph 3:20), but at least satisfaction. We serve an awesome God, we are not to *make-do,* and be complacent. *We do not serve an average God, so we should never settle for average!*

God has promised to supply my needs; (Phil 4:19) to satisfy me, with long life, (Ps 91:16), and give me *all* things that pertain to life and godliness, (2 Pe 1:3). If a craving tries to come upon me, I recognize it may be the *spirit of dissatisfaction*; I will not give in to it. I will not let it in, or let it have reign in my life. Instead of giving in to demonic suggestion, I will open my mouth and resist, by speaking the word of God.

Satisfaction is a gift from God; the gifts of God are not for Satan and his kingdom. If a demon has been in existence for 2000 years, (for example), and has influenced 30 lives, and maybe possessed at one time or another, the other 10; and all of those people have eaten all the ice cream they could get into their mouths, and the demon still isn't satisfied; it will never be satisfied! Think of yourself for a moment; if you love ice cream, can *you* get enough? But with God satisfaction can be a reality.

Affirmations:

I bind, and cast out every Snack Demon, Dining Demon, Eating Demon, every FAT Demon, in the name of Jesus.
I loose the Spirit of God, Wellness, Health, and wholeness in my life.
God has promised me long life & Satisfaction, I am satisfied in Him.
I will finally obey my mother— I do not put things in my mouth that shouldn't be there.
I do not put things in my system that are not therapeutic, or I do not put there permanently.
My system is clear of sin, by the blood of Jesus.

Soul Cravings

After all that eating, the craved food is still a mystery. If you knew what it was, you could get it. But you don't know what it is; it's not ice cream, it's not pizza. It's not a *natural* craving; it's a **Soul Craving.** A craving of the soul cannot be satisfied with food. You may think you know what you want, or what you crave. You may have that thing, only to be disappointed to discover that wasn't what you thought you desired, in the first place.

> ... when an hungry man dreameth, and, ...eateth; but he awaketh, and his soul is empty: or as when a thirsty man dreameth, and, behold, he drinketh; but he awaketh, and, behold, he is faint, and his soul hath appetite: so shall the multitude of all the nations be, that fight against mount Zion.
> (Isa 29:8)

The soul has appetite, it hungers, it thirsts, it desires, it wants, it pants, it yearns to be filled, and satisfied. Appetite recurs. If it liked what it got, then it wants it again and again. If it doesn't like what it was fed, then it hungers, thirsts, desires, wants, pants, even yearns for *something else*. This is called choice and preference.

Your soul is comprised of your emotions, will, and intellect. Emotions want and need to be satisfied. Love is an emotion, for example, that wants to be returned. Intellect wants to be reflected. God made us for relationship with Him, and other humans. Soul desires that drive people to seek satisfaction, often have to do with relationships. When relationships are non-existent, or out of order, emotional needs may escalate to a *Soul Craving*. Something that is chronically lacking in the emotions, may show up as a *Soul Craving*. It could be a yearning so deep, that you believe that it's part of your soul, or your essence. You may believe that if you don't have it, you may die, or something *worse* could happen to you.

A *Soul Craving* could be the result of a physical, or flesh desire that has been so long-lasting, (chronic); and you have thought on it so long, and so often, it's part of your life. You live for it — or believe you do. (**Oh, if you would study the Bible like that!**) It's like a raging thirst, or driving hunger. You think on it the first thing in the morning, the last thing at night, and then you go to sleep, only to dream about. You talk about it to anyone who will listen. You now believe you must have this thing at any cost, or that life just won't be worth it; this is a *Soul Craving*. It could be goal, a success, an object, such as a sports car, a career, a person, a relationship; anything! It could be anything you want, or believe you want, or anything you think will make you feel satisfied, complete, or happy. A *Soul Craving* can lead to obsession.

Flesh Cravings

*A*nd the mixt multitude that was among them fell a lusting: and the children of Israel also wept again, and said, Who shall give us flesh to eat? (Num 11:4)

The flesh is not part of the emotions, but when emotions are not satisfied, there can a spillover of want, or need in the **flesh**. Ever notice people who don't feel successful may overeat, or people who don't feel fulfilled in other areas of their personal dealings may drink, or have other vices. People who don't feel loved may take on bad physical habits. These people are appeasing their craving with something for the flesh, to try to satisfy, or cover up an emotional, (soul) need. These *Soul Cravings* have been misdiagnosed, and mistreated as flesh needs or problems.

Sexual frustration, for example, may manifest in a *Soul Craving*, where the person is obsessed with finding a mate. They may not be looking for a mate at all, just sex. Loneliness may manifest the very same way, a person may feel unfulfilled in personal relationships, or friendships; there may be nothing sexual about it. When the *Soul Craving* presents, the person may try to satisfy it with something physical. Food, alcohol, drugs, or sex, are common mistaken substitutes. There are no *natural* substances to satisfy a *Soul Craving*. But in trying to satisfy it, a Flesh *Response* may occur. A person may tie those two things together, and believe the Flesh Response is the indicator that the *Soul Craving* has been satisfied. It may not be, at all. If it's not, the *Soul Craving* urge will arise again, and again. When it arises, a person may set out to recreate the same experience, trying to satisfy it again. (This has now become a flesh addiction.) This may explain why so many people who get married just to satisfy a *Soul Craving*, may marry the wrong person, but find they are still not satisfied being married.

Good News! God has promised to satisfy us, so that we do not want. We should be free of the torment of Soul Cravings for tangible items, and even emotional things such as Love, and relationships. We should have **all things** that pertain to life and godliness, in abundance, not just barely enough.

> If we are to have a *Soul Craving*, it should be for God, and the things of God.

**As the hart panteth after the water brooks,
so panteth my soul after thee, O God. (Ps 42:1)**

Panting signifies thirst, or extreme desire. Our spirits are saved, forever out of the reach of the devil; but our souls are still exercising, and exerting will, (we are still making choices). Too often, souls are yearning for fleshy, (physical) and natural, (earthly), things, rather than the things of God. As Jesus hung on the Cross for us; His soul craved, even panted for The Father. He craved God. He didn't ask for a last meal, not ribs, not ice cream, not a cigarette; He yearned for God.

We should not wait for hard times, or adversity, to pant after God. Seek Him now; don't wait. He will satisfy your needs, and your *Soul Cravings*. If that means satisfaction and restoration in your emotions, so be it. If that means satisfaction intellectually, so be it. If our souls have been torn, or damaged for any reason, it is up to us to recognize it, or trust someone else who recognizes it, then seek God for restoration.

Sometimes that thing that is missing in many lives, that results in *Soul Craving*, is ***Jesus***. This is why people put too much emphasis on another human's ability, or responsibility, to make, or keep them happy. This is why some have an unrealistic view of what they can, or can't do for others, or what others can, or can't do for them, in relationships. Their *Soul Craving* is for Jesus, but they haven't realized it yet. In relationships, don't try to get from a man, or a woman, what you can, and should be getting from God.

The LORD is my shepherd; I shall not want. (Ps 23:1)
He restoreth my soul: ... (Ps 23:3)

That means I shall not want for any good thing. If I abide in Him, I'll just ask, (John 15:7), and He will give it to me. I shall not want. And, as I abide in Him, it also means I shall not want things that I shouldn't want, such as food, drugs, alcohol, and illegal or perverse sex. Not wanting, doesn't just mean I will not have to do without. It also means that I will not have a desire for ungodly things, because I am *abiding in Him*. But if a *Soul Craving*, or even a *Flesh Craving* tries to come upon me, I can resist it; because *I don't want it.*

The *chronic dissatisfaction demon of the spirit of whoredoms* is a **FAT Demon**; it can cause major eating, and overeating. You may find yourself *almost* satisfied, but then one little complaint may arise that voids the entire pleasant experience. That's a *spirit of dissatisfaction*, with a *complaining spirit*. That spirit, or both those spirits together, may be covered up by a person who is saying, *"I am discriminating, I have good taste, I am a connoisseur —I really know my .... food, wine, or (whatever)".* That same person that is never satisfied, or happy with anything. Don't get frustrated with them, pray for them. Because they are really, suffering from the *spirit of dis-*

satisfaction. We've got to bind it up, and cast it out, in the name of Jesus. And since it is bold enough to present itself over and again, we have to keep resisting, in the name of Jesus.

Are the Flesh (natural), and *Soul Cravings* the same thing? No. The *Soul Craving* can create a Flesh Response, and a Flesh Craving, *and* a Flesh Addiction. That's substituting a Flesh Response such as food for something that is missing emotionally, intellectually, even physically, or spiritually.

Trying to satisfy the *Soul Craving* improperly, may lead to the creation of fat, and all of the emotions that go with fat. Fat doesn't just happen, but when it becomes evident, the consequences to your body and mind, may show up in relationships as unrequited love, unfulfilled desires, dissatisfaction, or missed opportunities. Those emotional deficits, if long-lasting, may lead to one, or more *Soul Cravings*. To summarize, *Soul Cravings* can beget Flesh Cravings, **and other** *Soul Cravings*.

But the Flesh Craving can also create a *Soul Craving*. If the fleshly desire is denied long enough, but thought on, and planned, but unfulfilled, a *Soul Craving* may result. Sometimes the desire *cannot* be fulfilled, because the desire, or perceived need is for something that is impossible to have. Many times it **should not** be fulfilled, because it is a temptation from the devil. Without God, the Flesh Craving can persist to a *Soul Craving*. With God the desire can be resisted, and the cravings can be defeated, in the name of Jesus.

How can you know the difference between a Soul and a Flesh Craving? The Word of God. That's right, the Word of God.

For the word of God is quick, and powerful, and sharper than any twoedged sword, piercing even to the dividing asunder of soul and spirit, and of the joints and marrow, and is a discerner of the thoughts and intents of the heart. (Heb 4:12)

The Word of God has everything you need, and everything necessary for what ails you. The Word of God will divide what is of the soul, from what is of the spirit, from what is of the flesh. The Word will discern the thoughts and the intent of the heart. What do you want *from God?* Is it spiritual? Is it soulish, (emotional; are you in love, lonely, or broken hearted?) Food cannot satisfy any of those emotions. Is it fleshly, (are you in pain, cold, tired, or sick? Food satisfies hunger. Is that on any of these lists? Then don't use food *by mistake.*

If you ask, *What do I want?,* and look around you in the natural, you're sure to find — *food.* Instead, ask *what do I want, or need from God?* When you just ask yourself, you may not get an answer, or you may get a wrong answer. You may only know that you are missing something, or you want something, and it's making you feel uncomfortable. And you've been trained by Mom to eat for comfort.

But when you ask God, He is faithful to answer you, and supply it. If God's got it, then you know it's okay to receive it, (in His timing). If God doesn't have it, then you know it was a temptation. For example, if you ask for Sister Sonya's husband, to be your husband — God can't get that for you. That's a *Soul Craving* for a husband; you must be desperate. If you ask God, instead of asking yourself, or Sister Sonya's husband, if he wants to be with you, instead of staying married to his wife, then God can provide your husband to you. First He will help you make that temptation go away, if you let Him. Then God and you can address your soulish needs, and your emotional or physical needs.

But another emotion called frustration is working all the while you are confused about what you want, or need. *Frustration*, and *confusion* are **FAT Demons**. They cause you to reach for food. All this because you don't know yourself, your needs, and what you really want. Stop this cycle! Solve this problem by asking God, and applying His Word to your life's issues.

The Word of God evaluates the thoughts and intent of the heart. Acknowledge God, and He will direct your paths. He will help you through your struggle, so that you enter into a Rest from struggling.

> Take my yoke upon you, and learn of me;
> for I am meek and lowly in heart:
> and ye shall find rest unto your souls.
> For my yoke is easy, and my burden is light.
> (Matt 11:29-30)

The Lord has promised to restore our Souls. He will give rest from burning, and raging desires for things that bring torment, *either from having, or not having.* Those things could be anything from the torment of not being fulfilled in relationships, to the torment of the bondage of sin.

Affirmations:
I reject *Soul Cravings*, the Lord Restores my Soul.
I take the Lords yoke,
and His burden which is light.
I reject Flesh Cravings.
I am Spirit-led. I am not led by this flesh;
(no matter how much flesh I have).
I stir up my gifts, I build up my spirit,
I increase in God, so my flesh man is not bigger
than my spirit man.
From now on, I will STOP and Think
before eating —
Do I want this food? Am I hungry for *food!*

Am I using food to mask something else
that's bothering me?
I Promise —
1. I will spend time in prayer and meditation
asking God to show me my *Soul Cravings.*
2. I will seek to know why, I may have *Soul
Cravings.* I will seek to know
what is truly missing in my life.
3. to ask, and He will Satisfy me, and Restore my
Soul, in the name of Jesus.
4. I will have control and possession of my Soul,
and I will serve God with my whole self,
Spirit, Soul & Body.

Other "Eating Spirits"

Spirit of Bondage

There can be emotional bondage *(Soul Craving),* or flesh bondage, (physical craving) to eating, or an environmental bondage, one of habit; called Tradition. There is nothing wrong with the soul food tradition, for example, but a steady diet of soul food, never trying anything new, or healthier, is bondage. Not just food, but any tradition can be a form of bondage, such as having a martini after work everyday.

That holiday food craving, for example, isn't just a food craving, it's also emotional. Wanting to recreate the *emotions* of the past holidays, when *grandma was still here,* or *when we were young*, is more of a soul desire than a flesh desire, therefore it can't be done. **Food is <u>material</u> and emotions are not; therefore food can not satisfy emotions.**

If being in love takes your appetite, then you weren't hungry for food, you were *"hungry for love".* The need to have, or express the emotion of Love, was a *Soul Craving* that you had been covering up, or trying to satisfy with food. If having sex, takes your appetite, you weren't hungry — your flesh was craving attention and pleasure. That is a Flesh Craving. It is up to you to:

- Know yourself, (what do you want, and why?) Apply the Word.
- Discipline yourself, (don't give in to everything you think you want, no matter why you think you want it).

If the people part of a holiday experience can be recreated with food, then you didn't need grandma anyway. See how ridiculous that is. The reality is that the food didn't make the occasion; the grandmas made the food. If we miss Grandma, then let's say so, and remember her fondly in our hearts, our emotions, and our conversation. Those smells and tastes that you remember, and associated with *home*, will not bring back youth, or loved ones.

Untie the food from your emotions.

"Soul Food" was a movie about the sense of family fostered by making and eating dinner together. But quality family time could be raking leaves, or riding bikes to-

gether.   Cooking and eating together, was *their* family
tradition.   In the movie, no one talked about the fat
gained from eating. Like those Sunday, soul food din-
ners, other eating traditions present over and over to
tempt: Christmas, Thanksgiving, birthdays, just to name
a few. The bondage of a bad, or unhealthy eating tradition is a **FAT Demon**.

Because *mom* made chitterlings and pigs feet New
Year's Day, doesn't mean you have to, especially when
you have information about cholesterol, fat and calories.
That's the way we've always done it, doesn't have to apply to you, or me. God says to behold, He will do a new
thing. Soul food eaters, behold, I can do a new thing,
too, and so can you. Junk food eaters, behold, you can
do a new thing. Bad eaters, poor eaters, habitual *snack-
ers:* the new thing awaits you, too. You might become a
vegetarian, just because you can. Using wisdom to start
a new, or healthier tradition, doesn't disrespect your
Grandma. You can break free!

Affirmations:
I untie Food from my emotions.
I separate Flesh (physical) Desire from my emotions
by applying the Word.
I break free of unhealthy eating traditions!

Spirit of Addiction

*W*hat's the difference between a chocolate addiction, and a drug, alcohol, or sex addiction? They are all addictions. Addictions do not please God. The devil may want to introduce addictions to you in a subtle and likeable way; he may start with *food*. A food addiction might start with a simple family tradition, then move into a bondage, (you can't have Thanksgiving without sweet potato pie). Then it may move into addiction. *"That pie was so good, we need to have it every holiday"*; then every Sunday —. You get the picture.

Maybe you say you don't have a food addiction. *What is your food history?* If you make banana pudding for example, will you eat the whole thing? Then don't make it! Every time you see chocolate on a menu, you've got to order it. I'll tell you in love, you've got a problem. A food connection to anything more than nourishment, and sustenance of the body, is dangerous because the devil may try to start with food, then add, or substitute other things to entice, or entrap you.

For example, many people who smoke didn't pick up the first cigarette planning to develop a habit, or an addiction. Many smoke after eating, or in some cases, *instead* of eating. Addictions can start so innocently, but ruin, and take lives. Visit the ICU, (intensive care unit), of any hospital, and look at the patients dying because of devastating, life-long addictions; and many of those addictions were food, or food-related.

Where is the wisdom in creating the *habit* of consuming a chocolate *diet* milk shake instead of a meal, for several days or weeks, to lose weight. It seems that a craving for chocolate-flavored milk shakes will result. And if you give into it the weight will be put back on. *How do you shake that habit?*

Desire for food can start as a craving, then persist into addiction. To justify addictions, obsessions, poor eating, laziness, and bad behavior, people say, *"You have to die of something."* **No you don't**. Read your Bible; *you don't have to die sick*. You can get *called away* because it's your time. Psalm 91 says *"with long life, I will satisfy him..."* That means I can live as long as I want to; and healthy at that! I can live until I'm satisfied, and that is what I am doing! You could get raptured— **you don't have to die of an illness or disease, accident, or disaster.** But I have to *choose* to live! Sin is death, and righteousness is life. I choose to live! You must make your choice, too. Choose Life! (Deut 30:19)

> **I don't have to die of anything –
> to the Glory of God!**

Are food addictions, if they don't kill, the forerunners of addictions such as sex, drugs and alcohol? Are they the tricycles of more *dangerous* addictions, which are the bicycles and motorcycles? Could be. I don't know as well as you do. Has your food, (or other) addiction gotten worse, or better over the years? You can tell if you are becoming addicted to more, or fewer foods than when the addiction first began...and if the frequency of usage has increased or decreased. Have other addictions been added? Don't you think it's time to break that *spirit of addiction* that's running, or ruining your life? Use the name of Jesus; because at the name of Jesus, *every* knee will bow, (Philippians 2:10)

Addictions can go away all at once, with God's deliverance, and strong resistance, or taper off with discipline. You've heard people say, "*I used to love pizza, now I just can't stand it*". The addiction either went away, or into remission, or was replaced with something else.

Addiction remission? Sure. Maybe your addiction isn't active right now. You've seen people put down cigarettes for weeks, months, or years, and then suddenly pick them up again. That was *addiction remission*. It's a trick of the enemy, where the demon that influences the addiction doesn't rage like it once did. You may have prayed, and believed God for deliverance, and it may *appear* that you have been set free. But you may not really have deliverance. As long as you are not giving in to the demon's urges, then your health may be intact, but don't risk letting it take over again! Don't risk passing it on to your kids! Get rid of it! You need strong intercession, and spiritual deliverance.

A remission may be apparent if you conquered the addiction in the **flesh**, but not in your soul and spirit. That means you made up your mind to quit; you *decided* to quit smoking, for example, but nothing happened in your soul, or spirit life. So that spiritual influence, fleshly need, or *Soul Craving* drove you to begin smoking in the first place, still exists, you've just **decided** to ignore it. How long do you think you can do that? Or you may have already replaced smoking with something else — *like eating?*

Why should you care about the spiritual reasons for overeating? Because you don't want to just lose the weight; you want to **get rid of weight** (and burdens); you want to keep it off. If you lose the weight, instead of getting rid of it, along with what caused it in the first place, then you may *find* it again. Jesus, rebirth, and renewal must happen spiritually, since it is a spiritual battle. You can only be sure when it is bound up at the roots, and cast out in the name of Jesus.

Affirmations:

I bind up, and cast out the spirit of addiction,
in the name of Jesus.
I loose Temperance, Self-Control and
Spiritual deliverance in the name of Jesus.
I am not willing to lose anything else; in this life,
but I am willing to Get Rid of Excess Weights and
Burdens.

Spirit of Fear & Worry

*A*s mentioned, the *spirit of fear* can be a FAT Demon. It can freeze people in their tracks. In the natural
it can keep someone in the house, when they could be
outside exercising. Outside is where members of the fellowship takes walks. It's where the church plays volley-
ball. Fear puts on many different faces; fear of people,
and their faces, is spoken of many times in the Bible.
There could be a fear of playing in the game, dropping
the ball, or losing the game; the fear of letting others
down. That's why God says not to be afraid of their
faces — don't be afraid of *any* of the faces of fear.

The *spirit of fear* can immobilize, it keeps people
seated, when they should get up. It may keep you from
walking in the morning around the school tracks. Are
you afraid of the neighborhood dogs, cats, or *bugs*? You
may think that you're not going to lose any weight any-

way, so why go. That's the fear of failing.

The *spirit of fear* can bring on a case of nerves or anxiousness that may cause eating. Some seek *comfort food*, like chocolate, breads, pasta, and deserts, or a complete junk-fest buffet, eating everything in sight. Fear may lead to the *hand-to-mouth disease* of raising food, (with hand), to mouth, and eating mindlessly. This eating may accompany other mindless activities such as watching TV. The *spirit of fear* can add pounds; it's a **FAT Demon.**

Or maybe you *don't* overeat because of fear. But fear can freeze the digestive process. Some know it as heartburn, or gas; others know it as butterflies, or knots in the stomach. When you're afraid, the blood that is supposed to rush to the stomach to digest the nutritious food you've just eaten, is rushing to the extremities in *a fight or flight* response. Fear sends blood to the arms, and legs, (etc.) for running away, or fighting. This is why people who have nervous stomachs don't eat before a public, or major event. This is why people who get anxious speaking to crowds probably shouldn't eat before giving a speech. Depending on how gripping and chronic the *spirit of fear* is, it may mess up metabolism in a worse way than just gas or indigestion, and maybe permanently. Fear, causing improper digestion, and irregular bowel elimination, may work against you, to help the

FAT Demons. Improper bowel elimination can cause worse problems than fat.

That *spirit of fear* may have come from your mother as an infant. She overfed you, or fed you too often; she stuffed you, because she was afraid you were not getting enough to eat. And now you're used to full feeling; what I call stomach-conscious — can't sleep without it. That infantile overfeeding increased your brown fat cells, which predisposed you to being heavier in adulthood than you might be comfortable being. The *spirit of fear* is a **FAT Demon**.

Fear causes missed opportunities, jobs, career advancement, or ministry. Then because of it, on a secondary level, feelings of uselessness, defeat, self-loathing, and un-forgiveness may flood in. All of this, unchecked can lead to depression. Fear is a **FAT Demon** that can open the door for other **FAT Demons**, such as, the *spirit of depression.*

Worry

*W*hile eating, the mind is on the taste buds. After eating sufficiently, you become stomach-conscious. All the while, you are not thinking of your outside problem, are you? Have you noticed people who hum, sing, or wiggle their legs while eating? They have forgotten the cares of this world. Food has become an escape and a distraction for them. As mentioned earlier, eating can be a very real distraction. Always be spiritually alert. Worry and escapism, are only distractions, and they are **FAT Demons.** When you get through eating, the same problems will still be there. But if your weight increases because of the eating, then there are added problems.

Phobias

*F*ear is no small thing, and the devil really isn't playing with you. Little phobias should be overcome and cast out as soon as you are aware of them. No longer should you announce, *"I am afraid of...."* anything! That is a foothold for the *spirit of fear*. You need to overcome fears of everything from spiders to snakes, to cats to dogs, monsters, thunderstorms, dentists ....*whatever!* God has not given us fear, but Love, Power and a Sound Mind, (2 Tim 1:7) If you have the Fear, you don't have the other three. Would you rather have one bad spirit, or three good ones?

You might be saying, *"It's just a little phobia".* Good! It's an opportunity for you to work your little faith. The world tells you to accept yourself with your faults and weaknesses. But a phobia isn't a part of you — fear didn't come from God, so **you must reject it**. It's a foothold for the devil; a trick of the enemy; and this is war!

God says to cast down imaginations, He says, *"Fear not"*, over and over again in the scriptures. He says, "I am with you".

The first line of defense is Resistance. But you have even greater weapons against him than he does against you. But don't forget, the devil is spirit, so you've got to use spiritual weapons.

Affirmations:
I bind up, and cast out the spirit of fear, in the name of Jesus.
I loose the spirit of Love, Power and a Sound Mind.
I purpose to conquer every phobia
in the name of Jesus, to the Glory of God.
I resist the devil and he flees from me.
I untie eating from worry, Fears & Phobias.

Anger (Unforgiveness & Bitterness)

*U*nbelievers, or uncommitted Christians seek *payback* on the person with whom they're angry. *Living well is the best revenge,* but many people, (women, especially) go to the kitchen, for a box of Hagen Daz, or Ben & Jerry's ice cream, to plot revenge.

How many people have you heard say, *"I was eating everything in sight, and then the answer came to me!"*

None.   No one.   It's like those people who look up in the
ceiling for answers to questions; it's not there!   When
you eat, blood goes to the stomach for digestion.   In order to think, and plan, even if it's revenge strategy (not
recommending, unless it's against the devil), the blood
needs to go to your *brain*.   *Food cannot answer anger,*
there are no emotional answers in food.

Your momma taught you how to eat right.   Maybe you
have a strange desire to get back at her, or prove yourself grown up by eating all the things she told you not to
eat.   As a child, Ed didn't like sharing with his sister, so
now he eats whole, large bags of snack chips, in one sitting, just because *he can.*   This started out as a way to
fill a deficit he felt since 35 years ago, whether emotional, (did he feel unloved, jealous of his sister), or
fleshly, (was he still hungry), he doesn't know.   But now
the flesh has taken over.   He is addicted to snack chips.

It is dangerous when the emotions drive the flesh.
Emotion-driven flesh can influence anything from overeating, to crimes of passion.   At the very least, the *spirits*
of anger, un-forgiveness and bitterness are **FAT Demons.**

Did you catch that?   I am telling you that if you forgive
so and so, even for the horrible things that he, or she did
to you, that you could lose weight.   The pain and the hurt
of the past episodes in your life is a **weight** in the spiri-

tual and soulish realms. It may also be the cause of the weight that has manifested on your physical body. It's a burden. Forgive, stop hating, put away the bitterness; let those things go, and watch the weight go with it. You must get rid of those **FAT Demons**. They are clinging on to you by your emotional hurts!

<u>Affirmations:</u>
**Vengeance is the Lord's,
I don't need to plan revenge,
except to follow the Word of God,
and be active spiritually in warfare.
I don't need to eat because I am angry.
I untie eating from Anger.
I put away the works of the flesh,
such as anger and pride.**

Pride

*T*he *spirit of pride* can be a **FAT** Demon. Many fat people, especially those who have socialization problems, are overly prideful. They want to be right all the time, even if it means proving others wrong. It's a 24 hour a day thing for them. If they can prove another person wrong, they themselves won't look so bad, (they think). These people *eat*; they are inundated with the *spirit of pride* and *obesity*.

**They are inclosed in their own fat: with their
mouth they speak proudly. (Ps 17:10).**

God did not make a mistake in describing these people as being enclosed in their own fat. Literally they are
so full of pride and self-righteousness, that there is not
room for anything else in their lives. They are so prideful
that they cannot even forgive themselves for making mis-
takes — so they don't make any. At least that is what
they want to believe, and have you believe. They are so
emotionally wounded inside for feeling as though they
are less than perfect for past, and un-confessed mis-
takes, that they believe are hidden. They are unforgiving
of themselves, and others, so they eat, and eat, when
no one is looking.

Maybe you are not engrossed in your own pride —
yet. Maybe you're just a *little* prideful, you may be calling
it perfection. Maybe you mean well, and don't want to do
anything wrong. Perhaps you just get a little angry when
people accuse you of having done things incorrectly.
Perhaps it's a soul deficit, where your mom or dad con-
stantly criticized you when you were a kid.   Perhaps the
eating is a *Soul Craving* for reaching perfection, or getting attention, recognition, encouragement, or praise. As
a child, maybe your school teacher criticized you publicly, and embarrassed you. Now you want to prove them

all wrong by being perfect. Maybe you crave praise but when you can't get it, you may resent others, or try to discredit those who are very successful, or get a lot of attention and appreciation. *Pride* is a **FAT Demon.**

If you are the child of an alcoholic parent, you may have a real perfection problem — you could be running over with pride. Don't be embarrassed, the confession and release of pride can be a private act, entirely between you and God. Confession is the start to get rid of pride, this **FAT** Dining **Demon.**

(Children of Alcoholic Parents is a good book to read).

Affirmations:
I untie my emotions from food.
I untie eating from feelings of pride.
I put away the works of the flesh,
such as anger and pride.

Spirits of Shame, Guilt, Self-Pity
*A*ny of the sins that make you want to physically **hide,** or hide some aspect of yourself, physically, emotionally, or spiritually, potentially bring **FAT Demon activity** with it. I wonder if Adam and Eve gained weight after

sinning? **Guilt, Shame, Fear, Self Pity,** and **Depression** are all *Hiding Sins*. If you are under the oppression of any one of these emotions, then you may be influenced by a **FAT Demon.**

Dee picks up the staff lunch. One day the office splurged on burgers and fries. By the time the food got there, everyone was very hungry, because it was after 2 pm; so they started eating like lumberjacks. Dee nibbled. Feeling all eyes on her, *(although none were),* Dee blurted out, *"I already had a combo in the car, I didn't want you to see how hungry I was!"* Dee was having *twice* as much food as everyone else, but we all thought she was eating the same, or less. Dee was hiding food; and being heavy, she was hiding her true self. These *spirits of guilt and the spirit of gluttony* are **FAT Demons.**

Shame is a **FAT Demon.** Some people have endured horrible pasts, and don't want to be attractive, on purpose. With the help of their Eating, Dining, or Snacking Demon, they gain weight because of shame, to cover up the beauty that God intended them to have. They think they are hiding behind their heaviness. Usually these are such pretty and attractive looking people anyway. They have a beautiful presence and good hearts. They will find themselves attracting people anyhow, but not feeling comfortable doing so.

That light that God put in you, cannot be hid. Even

though there are **FAT Demons** trying to help you hide, and enclose what God put in you; it cannot be hid. **Get back, FAT Demon! Ministry is coming forth**, and the child of God will be happy, healthy and comfortable too!

Affirmations:
I untie my emotions from food.
I untie eating from feelings of shame, guilt and
other emotions that make me want to hide.
I put away the works of the flesh,
such as anger and pride, guilt, shame and fear.
I put on the Holy Spirit of God
With Power, Love, and a Sound Mind,
with Forgiveness and Self Control.

Spirit of Infirmity

*N*ot everyone who is infirm or sick, is heavy or fat. Some small people are sick because they *can't* gain weight, (we are not talking about them in this book). The reason I call the *spirit of infirmity* a **FAT Demon**, is because of the sympathy sick folk get. When adults feel sorry when children don't feel well, they feed them. Kids get candies, snacks, sodas, and other foods to *cheer them up*. If food can cheer you up, then we all ought to be pleased as punch. Children often get a burst of energy after eating; they may want to get down from the table and dance around, or run and play. But that energy surge is from the increase in blood sugar levels; not from being *food-happy*. I've never had a food to make me happy — energized, yes; but not happy. Ask any depressed person which food makes them un-depressed, and they will tell you — none. They make counseling, medicine, and God has prayer and deliverance for your depression, not food!

Sympathy feedings can fatten up a patient. Then the patient is miserable, and other emotions may flare up. Don't overfeed yourself, or your child in the attempt to be *cheered up*.

Alcohol toasts also boast the word, *Cheers!* Alcohol is a mood elevator (first), then a mood depressor. Alcohol can really put on the pounds —it's a **FAT Demon**, too. It can't cheer you up any more than food can. A lot of the time the food that you enjoy, and have been eating, is what has made you sick in the first place. Food can be a weapon of the devil's warfare.

Another way the *spirit of infirmity* may cause weight gain is the secondary effect of many prescription medicines. Steroids, for example, can really cause quick, and dramatic increases in size. Marge, a petite young woman, was a size 4 at the beginning of summer, suddenly was a size 16 at the end of the same summer, and she was only 4'9".

A lot of medicines cause discomfort, so you may be eating just to settle stomach cramps. Some drugs and medicines, make you feel plain hungry, then eating is to satisfy real, or perceived hunger.

The Bible calls drugs sorcery. Those drugs that are mind-altering are more dangerous. During the time the drug is *working*, you may become more susceptible to demonic influences. When the drug wears off, suddenly, you're hungry.

I'm am not telling you to put down any life-preserving, or life-improving drugs; consult your own physician. Just know what your physical, and *spiritual* concerns will be from using certain drugs.

Affirmations:
I don't have to die of anything
I bind up, and cast out the spirit of infirmity.
I loose the Spirit of God, the spirit of wellness,
health, and wholeness in my life.
I use drugs therapeutically under wise counsel of
physicians, Dr. Jesus and the Holy Spirit.
I leave no room for spiritual influence that is
not of God.

Spirit of Divination-Sorcery

*D*rugs (sorceries), may increase appetites. Even therapeutic drugs, (prescriptions that promote healing) sometimes increase appetites, especially prescriptions that read: *Take with food.* A habit of taking medicine with food, (or food with medicine), when you might not need to, *just to be sure*, is a way drugs bring on weight. This is especially true of long-term drug therapy. The tradition, *Mom did it this way,* may lead to extra pounds piling on, or sick people get all the ice cream they want).

Recreational drugs can cause incredible cravings in many people. It's considered a joke to *munch*, or binge after using certain drugs, especially marijuana. Maybe while intoxicated, or *high*, out of control of the mind and body, a **FAT Demon** gained temporary control, and strongly influenced the user.

People crave food after *getting over* a drug, alcohol, or cigarette addiction. One can get over an addiction, but the *spirit of addiction* can persist. When Martin, who is unmarried, became saved, he gave up fornication and adultery, which he admits he used previously, for **entertainment**. He gave up sex, for God. But now he eats at least two pints of ice cream a day, to make up for it. Those sugar rushes make Martin silly, and giggly. But they give him the sense of feeling *happy.* He is using this particular food as a drug. The body is not designed for extreme sugar rushes, such as the kind that comes from sweets and desserts. This is dangerous to his system. Martin traded a sex addiction for a food addiction. It's the same spirit, different substance. Remember when you used to love ice-cream sandwiches, then a certain candy bar, then replaced it with another food. Food can be very addictive. What's more, it's legal, it doesn't cost too much, and it's easy to score.

Warning: Replacement addictions aren't always food for food. As in Martin's case, a sex addiction was replaced with food. The converse could occur, a food addiction could be replaced with a sex addiction. (Or something worse). Don't allow it! Take charge of your body, mind, and soul so you can be used in the Kingdom of God!

Maybe food was never a temptation to you until you got over that habit, (drugs and cigarettes, especially). If so, you've gotten over the *habit*, but not the addiction. You've still got work to do; you still need physical and spiritual deliverance.

> **If abused, *food* can be a
> mind & body-altering drug.**

Affirmations:
I bind up, and cast out all the works of the devil in
my life.
I bind up, and cast out the works
of drugs and sorceries.
I use drugs therapeutically under wise counsel of
physicians, Dr. Jesus and the Holy Spirit.
I leave no room for spiritual influence that is
not of God.

Spirit of Heaviness – Depression

*G*ot the munchies again? What will it be this time?

Depends on what's bothering you, doesn't it? If you're feeling depressed; you want something to *cheer you up*, like chocolate. If you're feeling happy, you might want to celebrate, and have some chocolate. If you're feeling sad about a relationship breaking up, you might want something that will make you feel better; maybe some chocolate. If you're mourning the loss of a loved one, you might want some real food like Mom used to make — some soul food. You might want to finish that meal off with some cake; maybe some chocolate cake. Sounds like you got what I call a Chocolate Demon; and it's not cute, funny, nor is it something to brag about. You've heard folks say it — gotta have my chocolate.

Who's gotta have it? You or the demon?

But the Chocolate Demon is not the only *eating de-mon*. Many of the other demons eat and encourage aggressive appetites. Depression, like some others named along with the spirit of heaviness can stir up the Chocolate Demon, causing many to eat, and overeat. It's the Flesh Response spoken of earlier, *(Soul Cravings, p. 87)*. Maybe chocolate made you feel better the last time you went through this, or something similar. Maybe mom always gave you cocoa when you were unhappy, or not feeling well.

Depression can lead to heaviness. You don't think God named it *heaviness* by mistake, do you? Heaviness is over-grieving. Where the normal grieving period might be six months or a year, a person who is under the bondage of the *spirit of heaviness* might still be grieving four, five, or 20 years later. They may have grieved their life away, as a perpetual victim, widow, or divorce'. Heaviness is much worse, and more escalated than depression. Both can lead to acute and chronic eating, especially if you're conditioned to reach for that *happy food* to fix up the blues you feel.

Affirmations:
I untie eating from feelings of sadness,
disappointment and depression.

I bind, and cast out all the works of the enemy in my life; depression, heaviness, and sorcery, in the name of Jesus.
I loose the spirit of Love, Power and a Sound Mind, In the name of Jesus.

The I Don't Care Spirit (Apathy)

*T*he I Don't Care spirit is part of the *spirit of depression.* Don't ever say that you don't care what happens to you. Even if you don't really care. By speaking that, it opens up a big, wide gate that lets in all kinds of demonic oppression. Even if you feel like you don't care today, don't say it — because tomorrow, prayerfully, you may not feel that way. Hold your peace.

A living body is very attractive to a spirit that's looking for a place to dwell. The spirit has it's assignment, and it's own agenda — which is *against* you. In the natural, if you knew someone didn't like you, was against you, or was out to get you, would you invite them to stay in your home? No. Would you tell them they could come if they wanted to — that you didn't care if they came or not? No. But that's what you're doing if you say you don't care. In the spiritual you've got to make the same decisions and declarations, as you would in the natural, or you could get any kind of spiritual house guests!

By saying you don't care — you risk being overtaken spiritually. That's why the Word says that you were either hot or cold. The lukewarm, *I Don't Care spirit* can be run over. Milk that sits out becomes lukewarm, and all kinds of bacteria and germs can grow in it. If drank, it can make a person sick. That same sour milk has all sorts of life in it, that you can't see, but if you take it into your body, it can cause big health problems. There are unseen spirits that may try to influence you, if you don't state what you will, and won't allow. Just as in the world, if you don't vote, a candidate will be chosen for you. The same applies in the spiritual; if you don't choose a side, one will be chosen for you. If you don't choose God, the devil will send whatever he can get into your life. Rebuke the spirit of *I Don't Care*. Spiritual ambivalence is an open door to the devil. Be hot, or be cold, but do not be lukewarm.

> **Don't ever *say* you don't care what happens to you, even if you feel that you really don't care.**

Regarding physical ambivalence: Have you ever thought about what **size** you'd like to be? Seriously? Do you care? Or are you just doing whatever, eating whatever, and letting nature *take it's course?* Do you feel that you have any control over your body? Your life? Ambivalence, and I don't care, will create **whatever**. Decision will create what you want, something really close to it; or *something even better*. Why don't you **decide** what you really want.

Affirmations:
I reject the spirit of apathy, in my life.
I care what happens to me,
I care about my spirit, mind, soul and body.
I choose what I eat, it is not chosen for me.
I choose what size I want to be,
it is not chosen for me.
I choose God. I choose the Holy Spirit
I choose Life!

Slothful Spirit

*M*aybe you're just plain lazy. You don't want to get up in the mornings. You don't want to exercise. You want to take a nap as soon as you eat. Metabolically, something could be wrong with you, or there may not be anything at all wrong with you. The *spirit of slothfulness* could be enjoying sleeping *your* life away for you. Get up! The *slothful spirit* is a **FAT Demon**.

Hair Bondage

Maybe you have a legitimate excuse for not exercising; your **HAIR**. (This one defied a category.) **Hair Bondage** is not a type of *weave*, or maybe it is. Maybe it's idolatry, vanity, or truly a bondage. It depends on why a person acts the way they do because of their hair. (This is cultural, so if you don't understand, ask someone).

Those in Hair Bondage don't exercise, or don't exercise regularly, because of elaborate, and often expensive hairdo's. I struggled with this one myself. Whether to fully exert oneself in regular exercise, or preserve the $30-$70, sometimes $100 hairdo was the question. Did I want to look physically good, and wear a pony-tail so I could exercise? Or did I want to look *coiffed*, taking my chances on what my body physique would become as it reflected my leisurely lifestyle.

The Bible says that we should not be vain, or overly adorn ourselves; our beauty comes from the Lord, and it comes from within. The Bible says that bodily exercise profits little, (compared to spiritual gain). Is that license to not physically exercise? No.

Folks in earlier days didn't have aerobics because just to eat and live, they worked on farms. Because they worked so hard; they didn't need exercise and gyms. Our grandparents, (and parents), could eat a lot of foods, and more food than we can today, because of their lifestyle. They needed more food to fuel all the labor-intensive farm work they did. We don't need that same food, or the same amount of food to go to the grocery store, or order from a restaurant menu, then sit down, and watch a movie. **If you're going to eat like a farm hand, then you've got to work like a farm hand.** Balance is the Challenge.

> **Eating farm-style food,
> while living a city lifestyle will lead to Fat.**

Affirmations:
I reject the spirit of laziness.
I thank God my body *moves,*
I move it with purpose, to keep it healthy,
and bring it under control.
I will eat the kind, and amount of food that
correlates to my Lifestyle.
I bind up, and cast out the spirit of ignorance, the
spirit of not knowing what to eat, when to eat,
and how much to eat.
I loose the spirit of wisdom in feeding and caring for
my body.

Spirit of Procrastination

*M*aybe you're not lazy. Maybe you're just going to do

it later, or tomorrow; exercise, eat right, go to church, put that idea on the market. Tomorrow would be a better day after all, it will be easier tomorrow. True, there is a right timing, and a right season for everything in the economy of God; but false, is the idea that the better time is tomorrow. God says, "**Now,** faith is..." (Heb 11:1). So everything is not best done later. *The spirit of procrastination* is a **FAT Demon**.

Affirmations:
I reject the spirit of procrastination.
Now faith is — I will do it Now!
When the Lord says move, I will Move!

The Late-Night Demon

*T*he Late Night Demon has earned a dishonorable mention. Go to bed! Staying up late at night does more harm than you think. It robs you of valuable, and needed sleep and rest. It robs you of productivity the next day. It affects your appearance, especially as you mature. Look at those dark circles, or wrinkles around your eyes. Go to sleep!

While you're awake, what are you doing? Anything important? You are probably watching TV, and thinking about what you're going to eat next: a cupcake, soda, or coffee, loaded with cream and sugar. *The Late-Night De-*

mon is a **FAT Demon**.

Your Momma's been telling you, and now I'm telling you — Go to sleep! *Take that out of your mouth, and go to sleep!*

God spoke to many in dreams in the Bible. God can finally talk to you when you're quiet, and sleeping. Go to sleep! You may be missing out on some spiritual guidance and direction. Go to sleep! I have prayed many times, and gone to sleep, to wake up refreshed, *and* with the answer to my prayers. Go to sleep!

The body is supposed to fast food for several hours. That's why the morning meal is a *break-fast*. This is designed by God. Don't violate it. Go to bed! Overnight (or oversleep), your human spirit is still. Oversleep, you are quiet in the natural, and *fasting*. When you awaken, God has spoken. If all those conditions are met — then you heard what God said! There is something to this fasting, isn't there?

Stop trying to *act like* a grown-up, and **be** a grown up; go to sleep! Discipline yourself with proper rest. Follow the natural laws of God.

It is vain for you to rise up early, to sit up late, ...
for so he giveth his beloved sleep. (Psalm 127:2)

Affirmations:
I will get my rest.

I will fast several consecutive hours a day
(oversleep; 8 hours is recommended)
I will be quiet to hear
what the Lord has to say to me, (1Thess 4:11).

The Crowd Demon

Everyone else is doing it, is not reason enough to start to do anything. Everyone else was drinking coffee in college, between classes. I didn't know where everybody went — then I found *The Coffee Room*. I was not raised with coffee in the house, and was never trained to drink it. Yet I would *pay* for a cup of coffee, that I didn't even want, and pretend to drink it, just to be where the crowd was, and to socialize. Wrong reason, wrong environment, wrong people to make friends with. But in my late teens, I didn't know that. After a while, I started drinking coffee — *sorta*. The same applies with food, cigarettes, or any other bad habit — you are probably eating some stuff now, that you really never wanted to start eating. You've got to resist the peer pressure.

Because everyone else is doing it, is probably more of a reason **not** to do it, than to do it. Jesus taught differently to the Multitude than He did to His Disciples, than He did His Favorites. Do you want to behave like the crowd, as the multitude does, or are you strong enough to stand out, when it means no one else is doing what's right? The crowd demon is a **FAT Demon.**

Good 'N Fat

Many folks think that fat is better, especially in babies; so they over eat, and over feed their children. Yes, fat babies are cute, but not necessarily healthier. But there are some good things in the fat *in you*. There is good fat to eat: some helps your cholesterol, for example. Some fats are *essential*, that means your body can't make them, you've got to eat them in your diet. There is good in fat; antibodies are in the fat. Antibodies help your body fight illnesses such as colds, viruses, and bacteria. People who are too thin, can find themselves sickly, sneezy, and ill more often than non-skinny people. So some fat is good. There should always be a balance. Experts report what is ideal based on special measurements and tests.

The Challenge is Balance

Being heavier than you should will cause your heart to overwork, among other adverse reactions. Carl died at the age of 30, of heart problems. He weighed nearly 500 pounds. The average man weighs 170 pounds; Carl was the size of three men. The heart works based on how much blood it has to pump, to how much body. His heart worked more than three times as much as it would have if he had weighed 170. So at age 30, he had over-worked a heart that could have (hypothetically), lasted him to age 90. For Carl, the Cause of Death might read, *Heart Abuse*.

Balance is crucial. The challenge is Balance.

Affirmation:
I reject false balance, it is an abomination to God!
I proclaim Balance in my life — physical, financial, emotional, everything that should be balanced Is, in the name of Jesus.

*(highly recommended: **"The Need For Balance"**, by Dwayne N. Hunt; single audio, or video).*

The Fat & Skinny Of It

Spiritual bulimia occurs from eating up the Word, then rejecting it; or not applying it, (for whatever reasons). Maybe the person next to you on the pew made you mad. The pastor's wife had on another new suit, *and hat!* Maybe you were already angry at your husband when you got to church. Blame it on anyone you want, God says it's when the Word falls among thorns, (Mark 4:7), that it is rejected, and no fruit comes of it, because of the cares, and distractions of this world. A person who may hear the word and reject it, is as a spiritual bulimic, and a spiritual anorexic; (frail, weak, and undernourished).

The above are two examples of spiritual disorders, just as binge-eating, bulimia and anorexia, can cause metabolic disasters. Isn't this world we live in strange? Every kind of fattening substance you can think of is offered, then you are told you that you need to be thin. Go figure.

Affirmations:
A false balance is abomination to the LORD:
but a just weight is His delight. (Proverbs 11:1).
I will delight the Lord,
as I balance every part of my life,
physical, spiritual, emotional, financial, and social.
I can do all things through
Christ which strengthens me.

The Discipline of Not Being Fat

At the feast of life, all manner of sumptuous fare is

presented to you. You are to use wisdom and discipline in eating. God told Adam & Eve *not* to eat of the Tree. The devil came in with the very first advertising campaign, (*or infomercial; we don't know how long he took to convince them*), and **presents** the same tree that's been standing there all this time. He highlights the fruit, tells them what it will do for them, he talks about how it's going to improve them, and make them better than they already are. (Like what, God didn't do it right the first time?) Ever since, the devil has been suggesting the menu, *even for Christians.*

Lust of the flesh, lust of the eye, pride of life, (1 John 2:16). The devil is using the same tricks. Why do you think that restaurants *display* the food they want you to order? Why do you think they have dessert carts, and dessert trays. They don't just tell about the sweets anymore, they bring it to you and let your eyes lust after it. It's the same old trick.

But there must be discipline; that's what defines a disciple. All manner of spiritual things are being offered to you, as well as natural things, yet you know which spiritual things to choose, don't you? You also know which natural things to choose; start with the discipline of food, the discipline of eating — the discipline of not being fat. It's something everyone can do. Romans 12 says it's your reasonable service. God knows you can do it, and

He expects you to. He expects you to present your body a living sacrifice, holy and acceptable. God knows there are temptations in the flesh life; James tells us that He does not give us greater temptations than we can bear. I believe God.

Paul says he keeps his body under, (1 Cor 9:27). Under what? Under control of his spirit, which is under God's Spirit. That is the man that walks by the Spirit and does not lust after the flesh. The lust of the flesh is what is pricked by the **FAT Demons** to stimulate the appetite, and cause the man of God to overeat.

The devil wants to take you out.
If that means *out* to dinner first, he'll do it.

Overeating may shorten the life span, lessen your ability to travel for evangelism, or impair your testimony. Perhaps you have the heart for dancing in your church's dance ministry — but you're out of condition. How does that glorify God? He knows your heart, yes He does, He knows that it's overworked from all that extra weight you may be toting around. An extra five pounds of weight, for example, requires an additional *mile* of blood vessels.

To be disciples of Christ, we can start with the Discipline of Food. Let's bless the Lord, and ourselves, in our eating habits.

Then there is the *ministry* of the discipline of not being

fat. What is that? As a teacher, preacher, counselor, evangelist, etc., you will tell, and show people what to do, and how to live their lives. As a Christian you represent God. Don't embarrass Christians by misrepresenting. Are you practicing what you preach? Or are you *not* preaching some things, because you don't live it out? Have you *limited* your ministry because of your lifestyle? If you do not have, and appear to have control over your own life, situations, body, etc., how will people receive you? How's your credibility? What will they perceive as your ability to guide, teach, direct and *exhort* them?

The Discipline of not being fat is a ministry all its own, and that same discipline will tremendously enhance your credibility, and ministry.

Affirmations:
As I am a disciple of Christ spiritually,
I am a mind disciple, I want the mind of Christ.
I am a disciple in my soul; He restores my soul.
Physically, I bring my body under control. My body, and my appearance, speaks to people before and after I ever do.
I am a delight to the Lord in Balance; False Balance is not for me, anymore.
My body changes to reflect my godly Lifestyle.
My Lifestyle changes to reflect my true commitment to God.

Prayer
& Fasting

Some only come out by **prayer and fasting,** that's why you starve a cold. Don't feed a cold, it will end faster. Take in clear liquids, and plenty of juices, the same things you would consume in a basic fast, and the cold will come out. Stay away from heavy foods and dairy products such as milk, and cream products, they produce mucous, (which is what you're trying to get rid of). God has cleverly inserted an 'involuntary fast' in with the common cold. What the devil meant for harm, his nasty germs and viruses; God meant it for good, (Gen 50:20). you can be *cleaned out* in the process of having a cold.

> **God has cleverly inserted an involuntary fast In with the common cold.**

Some only come out by **prayer and fasting,** (Mark 9:29). Spirits of addictions flee quickly with fasting, cigarette smokers, drinkers, lust and drug addicts have reports of good success when fasting *food,* **and** the addicted substance.

Is not this the fast that I have chosen? to loose the bands
of wickedness, to undo the heavy burdens, and to let the
oppressed go free, and that ye break every yoke?
(Isa 58:6)

**Some of the main spirits that come out by fasting
are the ones that influence eating.** If you don't feed a
stray cat; it won't stay at your house. If a Dining or
Snack Demon tries to influence you to eat, and you don't
give into it, it will leave. Even if you have given into the
Chocolate, Ice cream, Soda, or Snack Demon in the
past, if you start resisting now, it will flee from you. If you
don't think you can go cold turkey with *all* the snacks,
and foods, then resist the demons one at the time. Try
resisting, (fasting) the Soda Demon for a week, then a
month, then several months. Conquer it! Then move to
the Chocolate Demon. You can do it! I personally fasted
chocolate to prove to **myself** that I didn't love it more
than I loved God. Now, I can take or leave chocolate.

**Submit yourselves therefore to God.
Resist the devil, and he will flee from you. (James 4:7)**

The first time you resist will be the hardest; it may be
something like withdrawal from drugs, alcohol or cigarettes. You may get real physical symptoms; such as,
shaking, nervousness, jitters, anxiety, crankiness, or irri-
tability. But you can do it!

Think about your victory over food, what it will do for the rest of your Christian walk, think about your testimony, think about what it will do for your witness, and your ministry.

- If you can resist this demon, think of all the others that will flee along with it. (They like to travel in packs).
- Generationally, look at what it will do for your family, you won't be passing **FAT Demons** to your children.
- Think about the discipline you will achieve for your next victory. God will be taking you to the next level. Glory!

You are resisting the **FAT Demons** because you want to be obedient to God, and resist the devil. You want to be an over-comer, not an over-eater. If you're doing it for vain reasons, to be cute, to wear little outfits, to entice a man (or woman), it won't work. You must have the right motive, and the right heart. By not eating, you may actually lose weight — but the loftier, spiritual advantages may not be attained.

Affirmations:
I resist FAT Demons:
I fast to cause them to flee, to the Glory of God.
I break all generational curses in my family,

In the name of Jesus.

Spiritual Stream-lining

God chooses foolish things to confound the wise. Water is used to put out a fire; yet **water can burn fat.** Huh? Elisha built an altar for the sacrifice of bullocks, against the prophets of Baal. Elisha's altar had the sacrificial fat, *and* was doused with water, *but it burned anyhow*! (1Kings 18:33-38). That's God!

That's a spiritual point. In the natural, water is necessary to burn fat. If you were to study the biochemistry of the body, (which we will not do here), you would find that water is necessary for the breakdown of fat into energy. This is why water will help get rid of fat.

<u>Affirmations:</u>
I think, and I Drink — Water.
Excess weight, the devil's burden, is destroyed
because of the anointing.
I am anointed.
My body changes to reflect my godly,
and anointed lifestyle.

Water

*W*ater is mentioned in all 66 books of the Bible. If you inspired holy men to write a Bible, why would you have them talking about water all through it? Must be something to water.

And God said, let there be a firmament in the midst of the waters, and let it divide the waters from the waters. And God made the firmament and divided the waters which were under the firmament from the waters which were above the firmament, and it was so. (Gen 1:6-7)

God separated the waters above, from the waters below the firmament; above and below the *heavens;* there are waters in heaven.

Praise Him ye waters above the Heavens. (Ps 148:4)

And He showed me a Pure River of water in Life, clear as crystal, proceeding out of the throne of God and of the Lamb. (Rev 22:1)

This didn't make a lot of sense, initially, but since there was so much talk of water in the Bible, I knew it was important. Water is used in a number of different applications in our everyday lives. Water is used for baptism, which is a **covenant**. So God continues to **confound the wise**, by using something that can *dissolve* things, as a sort of **glue** that binds. (Matt 3:11, Mark 1:8, 10; Luke 3:16, John 126, 31, 33; John 3:5,, 3:23, Acts 1:5) Only God!

Water is used to wash with, to cleanse our external selves (skin), (Matt 27:24, Luke 7:44; John 13:5). It is said that when impurities, and sickness sweat out your pores, you should wash them away as soon as possible, to prevent them from going back in through those same pores, by simple osmosis. You'll be healthier, if you keep your external body clean. (And you'll keep more friends.) Doesn't it stand to reason that you can be healthier if you *"keep your insides clean too"*, (*quoted from Minister Erma Simpson, Basic Moves Ministry*.) There is also prosperity in water; remember the fish with the coin in it's mouth, Matt 17:27). God has put so much in water!

Water is used in (for) healing, in the Bible, *(see,* John 5:3-4, 21). When water was walked on, (Matt 14:28-29). Jesus asserted, and demonstrated His Sovereignty. He was as *Water from Above*, walking on the *waters below*. Jesus, being our Super Model, showed that we have dominion over everything, including the *waters below*, (earthly powers).

Water is a beverage or a drink in the Bible. (Matt 10:42, Mark 9:41, Luke 16:24, John 27, 9; John 4:7, 4:10, 13-15, John 4:46). Why would God have the Prophets and Apostles record something as mundane as the drinking of water? God is not mundane, and He is not trivial!

**The voice of the Lord is upon the waters the
God of glory thunderth; the Lord is upon many waters.
(Ps 29:3)**

God revealed what *Waters Above* and waters below meant. Water is spoken of in the Bible many times as Power, (John 7:38, John 4:7-15, John 19:34); and water *is* power. In the natural, hydro-power turns water wheels, propels boats, helps make electricity, and any number of other things. Spiritually, there are *Waters Above,* in the heavenlies; God and His heavenly hosts. But there are waters below, Satan, and his fallen angels. The *Waters Above* have power, and dominion **over** the waters below. When you, as a saint, drink common water, it becomes as *Waters Above*, because the Greater One is in you (1 John 4:4). The *Waters Above* "walk over" the waters below. Drinking water, as in fasting, flushes your system. Fasting drives out demonic influence, or oppression. Drinking common water washes out those Fat Demons that want you to drink sodas, and eat junk all day. They will flee.

The Bible tells the story of a man sentenced to hell, who wanted one drop of water, (Luke 16:24). He was in a dry place, where there was no water. This dry place was devoid of the Spiritual Water that we know that flows from the throne of God. This man thirsted, longing to be cooled. Yet, because of his sins, there was no water for him; not one drop.

Camels are the only animal species who can store up water for another day. We have to drink natural water, as we need it, while we can. We have to take in all the spiritual, and living water we can, while we can; so we will not end up in a dry place, with no water. The evil spirits of the devil are ravenous and scavenger-like, they are looking for dry places to land, dry places to rest.

When the unclean spirit is gone out of a man, he walketh through dry places, seeking rest, and findeth none. (Matt 12:43)

Biblically, a *dry place* is where there is no living water, where there is no Spirit of God; it's where there is no Word. An evil spirit cannot dwell in the house where the Spirit of God dwells. Notice I said, dwells, not influence. A Spirit-filled Christian can still be tempted, influenced, and can still make some unwise decisions. If you are an occasional church-goer, or only read your Bible on Sundays, a few verses at a time, (during the sermon, with the rest of the congregation), you don't have much Word in you—you are pretty dry. You can be tempted, deceived, and influenced. When tested, you can fail. Dining Demons, Snack Demons, and other **FAT Demons** can come in, *(among others),* if they choose. You don't have much resistance to them.

If you want to resist the devil, then fill yourself daily with *living water,* then drink plenty of natural water....and share....

And out of your belly shall flow rivers of living water.

For whosoever shall give you a cup of water to drink in my name, because ye belong to Christ, verily I say unto you, he shall not lose his reward. (Mark 9:41).

I used to think Mark 9:41 meant that God wants us to be *nice* to people; offer them a cool drink if they're thirsty. If you're a person that God needs to tell to be nice, then **be nice**. But people are thirsty for the Word of God, for the good news of Jesus Christ. That is the cup of water that you offer them. Great will be your reward in heaven, when you minister the Word to those whom you meet.

Jesus told the woman at the well, that if she knew who He was, she would have asked for Living Water, (John 4:10). People know you're a Christian. When someone asks you for living water, what will you offer them? When someone is hurting, needing peace, restoration, healing, and hope spoken over them, what will you offer?

Will you be in a hiding place thinking about yourself, and your own struggle with **Fat Demons,** or will you be there for them? That's also a strategy of the devil. If you're sitting around thinking about yourself all day being:

- Stomach-conscious, (How do I feel, what do I want?)
- Thinking about your weight
- Thinking about your size, your appearance
- Thinking about your social, financial, marital, personal situations, you will be:
  Depressed
  Static – no ministry can come out of you.

That's enough! It's time to come out of that place, and be what God has called you to be. Resist that devil, and he will flee from you, and you will be free to minister your testimony, and the Word to those who have a need, in season. It's time to be victorious over **FAT Demons**, and bring forth ministry.

For ye know the grace of our Lord Jesus Christ, that though he was rich, yet for your sakes he became poor, that ye through his poverty mighty be rich. (2 Cor 8:19)

In the above passage, Jesus became poor in what? Money, goods: what? What is the last thing Jesus said before He said, "*It is finished.*" He said, "I thirst", (John 19:28). Our Savior hung on the cross, bearing all the sins of mankind. God could not look on Jesus in that state, and turned His back on Him. Jesus became sin, so we would be sin-free. His Heavenly Father could not look on Him; He became poor in Spirit. He was without the Spirit; without POWER. He said, *"I thirst."* What did He thirst for? Not natural water. He had fasted 40 days to prove He could do without natural bread and water. But He yearned for Living Water: God, Our Father, Heavenly water, **Waters Above**.

Ho, every one that thirsteth, come ye to the water and he that hath no money; come ye, buy and eat.
(Isaiah 55:1)

Oh, people, **It's Free**. God is offering, and offering. You keep praying and praying, asking God what is the problem, *"Lord help me, Lord deliver me, Lord bless me"*. All through the scriptures, God kept sending people to Water, for restoration, for baptism, for drinking, for healing, for prosperity, for Life, for Thirst. Spiritual, Living Water is free. And He keeps offering over and over. Won't you accept it?

And he said unto me, It is done. I am Alpha and Omega, the beginning and the end. I will give unto him that is athirst of the fountain of the water of life freely.
(Rev 21:6)

DRINK WATER

Why do you think God is offering us so much water? Because there is Life in it. And it's so simple. A thing that we need everyday, a thing that is so commonplace, that all we have to do is drink, and it will bless us so much. It becomes what we need it to become. Take it and drink it! In underprivileged countries, or societies oppressed, among the first things to go are potable water, and freedom to practice their faith; ever thought about that? You've got both! *Ever thought about that?*

Water is Deliverance: Pharaoh and his army got drowned, in what, soda pop? **No,** water. God led His people out of Egypt, (a type of the world), even though the wizards had "powers", and the gods of Egypt had "powers", it could not match the Power of God. In their exodus, God parted the waters. He separated the waters of the powers of the world, from the waters of the powers of heaven. God is in Control. God has control of the waters, and He has given you dominion. He is showing you how to have dominion over the *waters below.*

The **FAT Demons** will persist if you don't drink water. The **FAT Demons** will take over if you don't take authority. Drown them! Drown them! Drown all of the devil's little Fat Army, just like Pharaoh's army got drowned!

Water is POWER. Did you know that man is more than 70% Water. You are more than 70% POWER! You are really full of what you need to live; so then shouldn't you be living a victorious LIFE!

Affirmations:
God is sending me to the Water.
The Water has everything I need, health, healing
Sight, quenching, Life, coolness, cleansing.
I think, and I Drink — Water —
the spiritual and the natural kind.

I'm Melting...

*W*hen water got on the wicked witch of the West, (Wizard of Oz), she melted. When water gets on your fat cells, it's as though they melt. Every time you drink water, think of all the **FAT Demon**-work you are destroying. Water is used in, and as *Deliverance* over and over in the Bible; let water be your deliverance from fat, and **FAT Demons.**

DRINK & THINK
DRINK WATER
DRINK & THINK

Maturing women, seem to gain more weight than men. It could be that they don't drink as much water as men. Ladies, just because you're all grown up, that doesn't mean you should drink all the cute stuff you served at childhood tea parties. The cute drinks, in the pretty stemmed glasses, with the umbrellas, flowers and garnishes, don't help; they hurt you.

Noticing the size of some coffee drinking–house guests, I purchased fat-free flavored creamers to serve them, and myself. None of the guests wanted it; they wanted the fat stuff; just the thing set aside for God. They also wanted four and five teaspoons of sugar per cup. (No one wanted de-caf either). They were drinking coffee to get flavored creamer, and sugar fixes. Bad news, these folks were addicted to coffee, creamers *and* to sugar.

Unless addicted to caffeine, sugar, or alcohol, the only reason you drink anything anyway is because you thirst. Or has the devil convinced you that you don't thirst? Has Satan convinced you that sugar, bubbles, hot coffee, or

flavored creamers *quench* your thirst? Of course not —
won't you accept God's offer to go to the water —

> ## *Drink Water.*

Rebuking The Devourers

> Bring ye all the tithes into the storehouse, that there may be meat in mine house, and prove me now herewith, saith the LORD of hosts, if I will not open you the windows of heaven, and pour you out a blessing...
> And I will rebuke the devourer for your sakes, ...
> saith the LORD of hosts. (Mal 3:10-11)

It's so simple. **Don't have the blues, when you've got the clues.** God says that He will rebuke the devourers for us. The Dining Demons, and the Fat Demons — they devour; and they cause you to devour. Snack, Chocolate, Ice Cream, Buttered Popcorn and Cola Demons, may all be part of *the Devourers.* Or you may be your own **devourer!** In the sense of eating, and weight. You may be *devouring* your own cash. Answer this simple question:

What do you spend your money on?

- Food?
- Clothes?

As the sizes change, the wardrobe must. Larger

clothes cost more money (more fabric). Are you paying more for your clothes than average-sized folk? You are your own devourer. Take back what the devil has stolen from you. Do you have a closet full of clothes that don't fit you, hundreds, maybe several thousands of dollars of clothes that you are going to get back into? Fight for your stuff! Get in shape, and wear your clothes, that the devil has stolen from you., Some people, actually have two, and three of the same item in their closets in different sizes. So when their weight does change, no one will notice — *they think.* A friend will notice, but a stranger won't care.

- Shoes

I bet you just love a nice looking pair of pumps, or sling-backs. But the more weight you put on those shoes, the quicker you'll wear them out. If you have to keep buying shoes because of weight, you are your own devourer.

- Fad Diets, and pills
- Exercise programs, equipment, and supplies.

Go to the cause, and stop messing around with the symptoms. Why are you eating?—spiritually? Remember that which is unseen brings into manifestation that which is seen. Are you doing it on purpose? What things can you do that you haven't tried yet? Have you addressed the spiritual nature of your life? After all, you are spirit.

```
DRINK & THINK
DRINK WATER
DRINK & THINK
```

God says He will rebuke the Devourer for our sakes and He will **pour out** blessings from heaven, (Mal 3:10-11). What is He pouring? *Waters from Above.* He's pouring out Power. Power to handle the situation, power to deal with things, power to trample over the enemy; power to bind up, and cast out the enemy. Power to get the things that pertain to life and godliness, and **keep** them. God is pouring out life-giving water, refreshing waters, from the throne of God; spiritual *and* natural water. God is showering us with heavenly authority, dominion, power, and blessings to use as we need.

What does money have to do with this? God says that you must be faithful in the little things, and He will handle the big things, (really, no pun intended). God will rebuke those **FAT Demons** for your sake, in the name of Jesus.

- Are you saved, and in the family of God?
- Are you water-baptized, in Jesus' Name?
- Are you Spirit-filled and flowing with Rivers of Living Water?
- Are you faithful in your tithes and offerings?
- Are you faithful with spiritual knowledge you've acquired? And to acquire *more* spiritual knowledge, or do you just want to know enough to *get by in life*?
- Are you faithful with the spiritual revelation that God blesses you with, including gifts of the Holy Spirit?
- Are you faithful with the natural gifts, talents, skills and abilities that God has blessed you with?
- Do you do, in the natural, as much as you can? Then you are ready for The Prayer.

Affirmations:
I pay my tithes to the Most High God;
I give offerings fit for a King.
He rebukes the Devourer for me.
I do not waste money on food, clothes, fads, diets,
exercise equipment or plans.
When it comes to buying anything:
I am Wise and Spirit-led.

(highly recommended: *Don't Refuse Me, Lord*, by Dr. E. Marlene Hunt.)

Bind & "Lose"

Maybe you haven't cast the Fat Demons out because you didn't know they existed, or that you had any, or that you needed to, or that you could. Maybe you were too embarrassed to ask anyone. It's a new day! Let's bind and loose in Fat Demon warfare. (Shall I say bind and "lose"?, pun intended)

Father, My Creator, Savior, and Redeemer. You are the Lord of the Universe, you are the Lord of my Life. I bless Your Name. Your name is Excellent, in all the earth; and the whole earth is filled with your Glory.

Father, if I am Spiritually Fat, I repent of it right now in the name of Jesus. If I have received spiritual information over the years and not shared it by ministering to others in need and in season, Father, forgive me.

Father if I have harbored revelation that you have imparted to me, and not released it according to Your Spirit, then I repent, and ask for Your forgiveness. I repent of not moving, not speaking when given a word of wisdom, a word of knowledge, a prophetic word, tongues, or interpretation. Lord I repent in the name of Jesus. If I have sat on the pew, with gifts, talents, skills and abilities while my church has done without, I am sorry and I declare this day that I will no longer be a bench warmer, when you have called me to be first-string.

If I have rejected your Word, after having heard it, as a spiritual bulimic, because of offenses and the cares of this world, Father, I repent in the name of Jesus. If I have not sat under the Word enough to receive a proper portion, as an anorexic, I repent in the name of Jesus and re-commit to being a good Christian, in right standing with You.

You said in your Word that if we confess our sins that you are faithful and just to forgive, and cleanse us of iniquity. Thank you, for forgiving me, and cleansing me.

Father in the name of Jesus I put away all works of the flesh, pride, anger, bitterness, idolatry, unforgiveness, shame, selfishness, guilt, I put away, in the name of Jesus all the works of the flesh, and instead proclaim that I will walk after the Spirit.

Where Spiritual Fat may have clung to me, I release it, I repent of it, I remove it now in the name of Jesus. Any eating disorder, or eating proclivity that is associ-

ated with any of these spiritual influences, I rebuke
and release also.

Where physical fat, as it may have manifested in, or
on my body, I reject it, I bind it up, and cast it out in
the name of Jesus — I keep only the fat that is good.

You said in your Word ((Matt 18:18), that whatever
we bind on earth will be bound in heaven, and whatever we loose on earth will be loosed in heaven. Father, in the name of Jesus I bind up, and cast out any
spiritual influence that has affected my appetite,
whether it be idolatry, excessive appetite, chronic dissatisfaction, pride, anger, guilt, shame, depression,
heaviness, infirmity, Soul Cravings, and natural cravings for excessive or bad foods, or anything ungodly.

I bind, and cast out whoredoms, sex sins, lust and
perversion, in the name of Jesus, I bind, and cast out
fear, selfishness, or any other emotional or demonic
oppression. I bind, and cast out sorceries in the name
of Jesus. I bind up, cast out, and reject the word of all
Fat Prophets over my life.   I renounce any negative
words that I have spoken over myself, and my body,
my being — Your temple.

I loose, in the Name of Jesus the Holy Spirit, the the
spirit of peace, a spirit of reconciliation, soul restoration, satisfaction, health, and balance in my body, a

spirit of selflessness, self esteem, forgiveness, Love,
Power and a Sound Mind. I loose, what You say
about me Lord — In the Name of Jesus, I thank You, I
bless Your name, Lord, as health, and spiritual right-
ness manifest in my life, I give You all the Glory,
Honor and Praise. Amen.

Affirmation:
Get Back FAT Demons!
Ministry is coming forth
in the name of Jesus!

To All Praise!

Minister Annette Jacobs —

A Praise leader who certainly has

"God's Stuff". Thanks for releasing

it to us all.

Thanks for all your

support help

the Fat Demons

Love Dr. Ma

Special Thanks

to

Pastor Dwayne N. Hunt
Sr. Pastor of Abundant Grace Fellowship,
Congratulations on Ten Abundant Years
of Pastoring, 1999!

AJ Praise
Min. Annette Jacobs, halalnike@aol.com

Basic Moves Ministry, Min. Erma Simpson
901-344-8892

Evan. Bonnie Chambers, Coral Springs, FL

Doretha Harris, Super-Duper Sister

Rev. Gayle Hunt
NetWorth Enterprises, networthE@earthlink.net

Prophet Kevin Leal, Pensacola, FL

Jackie McCreight, *Elegant Silks,* 901-344-9900

Kimberley Trice, owner of Braided Glory
901-346-7222 *(for freedom from Hair Bondage)*

Verneeta Williams, M.D.

r reorders of The FAT Demons, write, call, or fax, Grace Publishing.
line: www.drmarlenehunt.com
r Tape and Book orders for Pastor Dwayne Hunt, Call, Write, or Fax, Abund
ace Fellowship 901-789-GRACE , 1-877-88GRACE, Fax: 901-789-9376
line: www.dwaynehunt.com, or www.abundantgrace.org